School Counselors as Educational Leaders

JOYCE DEVOSS

Northern Arizona University

MINNIE ANDREWS

Northern Arizona University

Houghton Mifflin Company
Boston ▪ New York

Publisher, Lahaska Press: Barry Fetterolf
Senior Editor: Mary Falcon
Editorial Assistant: Lindsey Gentel
Project Editor: Kerry Doyle
Executive Marketing Manager: Brenda L. Bravener-Greville
Manufacturing Manager: Barbara LeBuhn
Manufacturing Coordinator: Priscilla Manchester

Cover image: Head Lantern in the Darkness, © Rob Colvin/Images.com

Printed in the U.S.A.

Library of Congress Control Number: 2005930907

ISBN: 0-618-56793-3

3456789-CRS-09 08

School Counselors as
Educational Leaders

CONTENTS

Chapter 5   Leadership Style Exploration   71

Chapter 6   Leadership Assessment   83

PREFACE

We believe that this is the first book to address leadership skill development specifically for school counselors. The book prepares school counselors in training to become effective educational leaders, advocates, and collaborators through exposure to current educational leadership and advocacy models and through active involvement in relevant skill-building exercises. The authors, a counselor educator and an educational leadership educator, have been involved with and greatly influenced by the National Transforming School Counseling Initiative led by the Education Trust (1997). School counselor educators who have been involved in this initiative have identified the need to better prepare school counselors for leadership and advocacy challenges in the schools.

The idea for this book came from the realization that although 21st century school counselors are expected to be leaders and advocates for children, they do not typically receive formal leadership skills training in graduate school. The authors piloted a leadership skills training program for school counselors; from what we learned in the process, we offer this book as a guide to other school counselor educators and supervisors as they prepare school counselors for their professional work in this new century.

Our goal in writing this book was to integrate a counseling and leadership theoretical foundation with practical principles and skills. We begin by describing the "new-vision" school counselor in the 21st century, the vision of the American School Counselor Association (ASCA) National Model, and the mandate for school counselor leadership. We familiarize readers with a number of contemporary leadership models that have influenced the field of educational leadership. We then identify and describe appropriate leadership assessment tools for school counselors and provide a framework for understanding leadership assessment results. Next we provide a format for incorporating each student's assessment results into the student's own leadership improvement plan. Throughout, we encourage students to engage in an ongoing process of seeking continuous feedback from others, self-monitoring, and revising the leadership improvement plan. We make readers aware of the leadership challenges ahead for school counselors and the importance of advocacy, collaboration, and data collection in addressing these challenges. We describe how school counselors can use leadership skills to design and deliver effective school counseling programs.

To enhance the learning experience for students, we begin each chapter with a case example of a practicing school counselor who faced leadership challenges in his or her school setting. Thought questions and further discussion follow each case example. Self-Assessment and Exploration exercises within each chapter provide students with opportunities to practice key leadership skills in the K–12 school setting. Review and Reflect exercises at the end of each chapter enable students to review the concepts in the chapter while reflecting on their own leadership qualities, beliefs, and practices. Finally, a list of Web resources relevant to the material covered in the chapter is also provided at the end of each chapter.

The ASCA National Model and the Education Trust emphasize the need for school counselor leadership training. We hope our colleagues in master's level school counselor training programs will find a place for this hands-on leadership-training workbook in their practicum, internship, and/or introduction to school counseling courses.

ACKNOWLEDGEMENTS

The reviewers of this text at the various stages of development provided many constructive suggestions that we incorporated into the book.

Thank you to the school counselor leaders from whom we obtained case examples to illustrate the chapters. We appreciated learning from the experiences of the school counseling graduate students who participated in the leadership training program we developed. We were inspired by the passion for school counseling demonstrated by the school counselor trainees we encountered in our classes and the professional school counselors in the field. Appreciation goes to Maria Buccilli, Margie Butler, Eric Emerson, Lerona Dickson, JoAnne Gellermine, Bruce Johnson, Brian Mathieson, Lynn Nystrom, and Zulema Suarez.

We thank Dr. Mike Miles and Dr. Ann A'Lee Miles, who graciously permitted us to include a brief version of their Leadership Behaviors Inventory. We thank the many leaders in the Transforming School Counseling Initiative for their tireless efforts in the past decade to give the school counseling profession a voice in educational reform. We especially thank leaders from the Education Trust, including Pat Martin, Reese House, and Stephanie Robinson, and leaders from the American School Counselor Association, including Judy Bowers, Mark Kuranz, and Trish Hatch.

Special thanks and recognition is owed to those who were instrumental in the production of this book. We acknowledge our colleague Jackie Duncan, who did two thorough reviews of the manuscript at different stages and made numerous useful suggestions that were incorporated into the text. Another colleague, Glynn Burleson, reviewed the manuscript in its final stages of revision with fresh eyes and insightful comments for refining the finished work. Mary Falcon, Senior Editor at Houghton Mifflin, worked closely with us on this project from conception to completion, keeping us on track to meet deadlines and advising us on revisions.

School Counselors as Educational Leaders

CHAPTER 1
School Counselors in the Twenty-first Century

A "NEW-VISION" SCHOOL COUNSELOR ENTERS THE TRENCHES

Zulema, a graduate of an M.Ed. program in school counseling accredited by CACREP (Council on Accreditation of Counseling and Related Education Programs), was hired as the new counselor at an elementary school in the middle of the academic school year. With other school personnel, she faced the task of helping the school overcome its "underperforming" status as designated by the state department of education. The counselor Zulema replaced chose to transfer to another school when she was informed that her position would be cut to half time. After the counselor left, a substitute counselor whose training was in teaching rather than counseling filled in until grant money was available to fund a full-time counselor. Zulema was hired with the grant money and saw an opportunity to demonstrate that school counselors can lead the way in making a difference in student academic achievement. She had learned about the "new vision" of school counselors as proactive educational leaders, planners, advocates, and collaborators who focus on whole school and systems issues and the academic achievement of all students. In addition, her graduate training had familiarized her with the American School Counselor Association (ASCA) National Model which incorporates the new vision of school counselor leadership roles. She was in one of the first groups of school counseling graduate students in the country to participate in formal training in educational leadership as part of their master's degree program. Zulema was eager to apply her learning.

Recognizing the need to create allies in the school, she quickly became acquainted with the principal and the faculty. To obtain a sense of their concerns for the school and their students, she surveyed them to determine the need for counseling programming. Initially she used the existing counseling referral process, but she soon saw the need for a mechanism to provide teachers with feedback. She revised the referral process and developed a form to give concise feedback to teachers concerning children they referred. Keeping in mind that effective school counseling programs are data driven, she became familiar with the district and school's data and noticed that her school's kindergarten had a high absentee rate. Out of a total of 121 students, 65 had absences ranging from one to three days, for a total number of 100 days during the month of January. This was the highest absentee rate of all grade levels at her school. She shared this data with her principal and her newly developed counseling program advisory team, and they decided to make attendance a priority at the school. The group consensus was to begin with a focus on improving the attendance of the kindergarteners.

In her first year at the school, Zulema complied with her administrator's expectation that she participate in student disciplinary sessions with the principal. Over time, however, she educated the principal and faculty regarding the ASCA National Model and best practices for school counselors that identify the most effective use of the time, knowledge, and skills of school counselors. By the beginning of her second academic school year, the majority of her time was scheduled for classroom guidance and groups. She provided weekly guidance lessons in each of the school's 23 classrooms and seven weekly groups for students in addition to her other school counseling responsibilities. This proactive approach to developing and maintaining a school guidance program resulted in a reduction in both referrals by teachers and demand for individual counseling sessions by students. Zulema developed a school counseling advisory council to assist with program planning and a detailed school counseling plan and schedule, integrating the guidance curriculum into the school's curriculum and customizing group offerings and advocacy efforts to student needs. Before the end of her second year as a school counselor, her school counseling program received recognition from ASCA for being a Recognized ASCA Model Program (RAMP) based on the National Model.

Case Discussion

Questions About This Case

- What were some of the key issues that this new school counselor needed to consider as she began her career as a school counselor educational leader?
- What other options might have been possible for responding to the unexpected assignment of helping with disciplining students?
- How can a school guidance advisory council support the mission of school counselors?
- What messages about school counselor roles and priorities does this scenario convey?
- What can we learn from this case example about working with the administration in a school?

Further Thoughts on This Case

Zulema is an example of a new generation of school counselors educated to meet the demands of K–12 students in today's schools. She was prepared not only with knowledge of the components of an effective school counseling program but also with the required leadership training that imparted the knowledge and skills to develop, implement, and maintain such a program. Even with the adequate preparation she received, Zulema found her first year as a school counselor challenging, and, at times, exhausting. She sought and found support from the district counseling department and other school counselors who strengthened her resiliency by encouraging her in her work.

This book is designed to assist in preparing school counselors-in-training and new counselors, like Zulema, to become effective educational leaders, advocates, and collaborators. School-counselor educators who have been involved in the National Transformation of School Counseling Initiative (NTSCI) of the Education Trust (1998), identified the need to better prepare school counselors for leadership and advocacy challenges in the schools. The approaches utilized in this book include exposure to current educational leadership and advocacy models and active involvement in relevant skill-building exercises.

CHAPTER OBJECTIVES

School counselors have served in a variety of capacities in public schools. Their roles have changed over time, in response to the changing demands of schools and the larger society. Because readers can review the detailed history of school counseling elsewhere, only a cursory review of the traditional school counselor roles is presented here.

The objectives of this chapter are to:

1. Provide a brief historical perspective of school counseling and its traditional focus as the backdrop to the transforming profession of school counseling today.
2. Present an overview of the current professional roles and expectations for school counselors as educational leaders.
3. Identify continuing challenges for professional school counselors and university school counselor training programs.

THE SCHOOL COUNSELOR IN HISTORICAL PERSPECTIVE

The development of professional school counseling over its history of more than 100 years has been influenced by a variety of forces. Noteworthy were the trends around the turn of the 20th century, including industrialization, immigration into the United States, migration from rural to urban areas within the country, and the concomitant exploitation of children. Additional influences on the emerging profession were the vocational guidance movement of the early 1900s and the development of the trait and factor theory.

In the 1940s and 1950s, significant developments occurred in the evolution of general counseling theory that affected the practice of counseling in all settings, including schools. At the same time, there were some rapid and dramatic changes in our country's national agenda with the commencement of the international space race. Resulting legislation had a major impact on school guidance programs.

During the latter half of the 20th century, school counseling emerged as a unique profession. By the early 21st century, leaders in the profession created a clear vision and a unified voice embodied in the ASCA National Model (2003), which established school counselors as educational leaders. School counselors had begun establishing an agenda for making significant contributions to educational reform.

Early Influences on the Profession

Approximately 100 years ago, during the Industrial Revolution, when American farming families began large-scale migration from farming to urban communities, the first publicly supported schools began to offer formal educational opportunities to people from all socioeconomic levels. These schools had diverse populations of students with all the associated challenges. School personnel, initially teachers, began responding to the need to provide students with information on occupational choices. School counseling as a profession later emerged from these early vocational guidance efforts.

Two early pioneers in vocational guidance were Jesse B. Davis and Frank Parsons (Schmidt, 2003; Sciarra, 2004). Davis was an educational and vocational counselor in Detroit, Michigan, and then later a high school principal in Grand Rapids, Michigan. In 1907, while serving as a high school principal, Davis began devoting one class period per week to student guidance. He is credited with developing and implementing the first systematic school-wide guidance program.

Shortly after Davis implemented his innovative approach to guidance, Frank Parsons, who was educated as an engineer but worked in several other professions as a social reformer and adult education advocate, founded the Vocational Bureau of Boston. Parsons' ideas about vocational guidance were described in his book, *Choosing a Vocation* (1909). The Vocational Bureau was established to target young people who were not attending school to provide them with occupational information. Parsons stressed the use of a scientific approach to career selection and included training vocational counselors as part of his plan for effective career guidance. Parsons' work greatly influenced a fairly rapid development of the school guidance movement in the United States.

In the midst of the school guidance movement, the National Vocational Guidance Association (NVGA) was founded in 1913 and first published what is now known as *The Journal of Counseling and Development* (Gladding, 1996). Shortly thereafter, in 1916, as a response to widespread exploitation of poor urban children, child labor laws and mandatory school attendance laws requiring children to attend school through elementary school were passed. Funding for public school vocational education came with the Smith-Hughes Act which passed in 1917, continuing the emphasis on vocational guidance.

The Use of Trait and Factor Models

The trait and factor model, first identified with Parsons, and later, Williamson, became prominent in the 1930s (Gladding, 1996). The trait and factor theory maintains that job satisfaction is closely correlated with matching personal traits, such as aptitudes and abilities, with job factors, such as needed skills and education. The armed forces were greatly influenced by this model and incorporated the use of standardized testing and measurement of military personnel starting with the two world wars. In addition, guidance counselors made it common practice to use tests based on the trait and factor model, adding a new dimension to their role while maintaining a vocational guidance emphasis.

Post–World War II Challenges

In post–World War II America, guidance counselors were challenged to respond to rapid societal changes that affected traditional values. These changes created widespread stress on families and individuals. Demand increased for mental health services and providers, and training programs expanded to meet the demand. At the same time, alternative approaches to the limited trait and factor and Freudian psychoanalytical approaches were developed.

Especially influential in the field of counseling was Carl Rogers's person-centered counseling model developed in the 1940s. This model contributed significantly to training approaches for mental health and guidance personnel and to the mode of delivery of counseling and mental health services. It was also revolutionary in that it challenged the trait and factor and the psychoanalytic approaches. The emphasis was primarily on individual counseling using a nondirective approach. Core conditions for a therapeutic relationship identified by Rogers (1980/1969) consisted of basic empathy, counselor congruence, and unconditional positive regard for the client. Person-centered counseling concepts continue to be valued and emphasized as fundamental in basic counseling skill training courses, including counseling practica and internships.

In response to a sense of challenge from the USSR's launching of the world's first satellite, *Sputnik*, the U.S. Congress passed the National Defense Education Act (NDEA) in 1958, providing funding for high school counselors in every high school. These counselors were charged with identifying gifted math and science students and advocating for them to attend college. The national agenda was for the United States to progress and achieve superiority over other countries in the exploration of outer space as well as in scientific and technological breakthroughs. In addition to providing for high school counselors, Congress made funding available to colleges and universities to develop school counselor training programs. The training programs in existence at the time reflected lack of research, consensus, and direction in school counselor preparation. The U.S. Congress made the funding available primarily to support school counseling as a means of advancing the United States in the space and technology race with the Soviet Union.

The American School Counselor Association

The establishment of the American School Counselor Association in 1958 identified school counseling as a profession separate from teaching. In 1962 (Cobia &

Henderson, 2003), ASCA identified the profession's goals, which included promoting personal development through individual and group counseling as well as vocational guidance and testing. Since the 1960s, the association has achieved greater consensus on appropriate school counselor preparation.

ASCA developed the National Standards for School Counseling Programs (Campbell & Dahir, 1997), which outlined expected student outcomes of comprehensive developmental school guidance programs in the areas of academic, career, and personal/social development. State departments of education establish minimum standards for professional school counselors but these are not always consistent with the standards of the profession.

The School Counselor in the Twenty-first Century

At the turn of the 21st century, educational reform once again became a primary influence on the evolution of the school counseling profession. For example, since 1996 the school counseling profession has been the focus of a national transformation movement initiated by the Education Trust. This organization actively promotes a new vision of the role of school counselors based on a social justice model.

In the early stages of the Education Trust's Transforming School Counseling Initiative, Reese House and Pat Martin (1998) outlined the new vision of the school counselor role and compared it with the traditional role of the school counselor. The new-vision school counselor was expected to be a proactive leader, committed to excellence in education and equal access to postsecondary education for all students. The school counselor was envisioned as an assertive advocate and social activist on behalf of students, parents, schools, and the school counseling profession. The Education Trust (1998) defined school counseling according to the new vision:

> ...a profession that focuses on the relations and interactions between students and their school environment with the express purpose of reducing the effect of environmental and institutional barriers that impede student academic success.

Table 1-1 illustrates the Education Trust's (1998) comparison of its new vision of school counselor roles and the traditional roles of school counselors.

In an effort to assist school counselors in defining their roles more clearly, ASCA adopted position statements regarding the profession. In one statement concerning the use of personnel without school counseling credentials, ASCA (1999) emphasized that school counselors should be leaders in creating, organizing, and implementing school counseling program activities for both credentialed and uncredentialed personnel. Currently, good graduate training programs prepare school counselors to participate in leadership in their schools. In addition to the position statements regarding the profession, ASCA (1999) developed a role definition for professional school counselors that provided greater clarity not only for school counselors but also for those with whom they work.

> The professional school counselor is a certified/licensed educator trained in school counseling. Professional school counselors address the needs of students through the implementation of a comprehensive, standards-based, developmen-

Table 1-1   The New Vision of School Counseling

Traditional Role Descriptors	New-Vision Role Descriptors
Mental health providers	Academic achievement promoters
Individual students' issues	Whole school and system issues
Clinical focus on deficits	Academic focus on strengths
Provider of 1-1 and small groups	Leader, planner, program developer
Primary focus—personal/social	Primary focus—academic success
Ancillary/support personnel	Integral educational team members
Loosely defined responsibilities	Focused mission/responsibilities
Record keepers	Data users for change agenda
Sorters, selectors for placement	Advocates for inclusion of all
Isolated or work with counselors	Teaming and collaboration
Guardians of the status quo	Agents for change and equity
Involvement primarily with students	Involvement with all stakeholders
Little or no accountability	Accountable for student success
Dependence on system's resources	Brokers of school/community resources
Postsecondary planners for few	Champions for all students

Adapted from the Education Trust, 1997.

tal school counseling program. They are employed in elementary, middle/junior high, and senior high schools, and in postsecondary settings. Their work is differentiated by attention to age-specific developmental stages of student growth, and the needs, tasks, and student interests related to those stages. School counselors work with all students, including those who are considered at-risk and those with special needs. They are specialists in human behavior and relationships who provide assistance to students through four primary interventions: counseling (individual and group), large group guidance, consultation, and coordination (p. 1).

Comparing Traditional and New-Vision School Counseling

This exercise provides an opportunity to explore the contrast between traditional school counselor roles and new-vision counselor roles in responding to the same situation and to examine and compare potential outcomes.

In small groups, discuss traditional school counselor roles versus new-vision roles and the different behaviors that might be exhibited by the traditional versus the new-vision counselor in the following scenario. Refer to Table 1-1 for the different roles. Make notes for reference in the spaces provided as you complete this exercise and as you continue to read and complete the exercises in this book.

Scenario: Because of Coronado Elementary School's poor attendance and academic performance records, the local and state school boards have a mandate to improve student achievement and attendance in the school. It is supposed to be a whole-school effort.

a. How would the traditional school counselor respond? What would be the role of the traditional school counselor, if any, in addressing this problem?

_____

_____

_____

_____

_____

_____

b. How would the new-vision school counselor respond? What would be the role of the new-vision school counselor in addressing this problem?

_____

_____

_____

_____

_____

_____

c. Which approach to school counseling do you believe will best serve the students and the school? Provide your rationale.

_____

_____

_____

_____

_____

_____

The ASCA National Model

ASCA described the work of school counselors in the ASCA National Model (2003): "School counselors help students focus on academic, personal/social and career development so that they not only achieve success in school but are prepared to lead fulfilling lives as responsible members of society." The four components of the comprehensive school counseling program are identified on the ASCA website: program foundation, delivery system, management system, and accountability. The vehicles for delivery of school counseling programs are the guidance curriculum, individual student planning, responsive services, and systems support. The emphasis is on preventive and developmental counseling to help all students understand and gain necessary life skills to cope with social, behavioral, and personal problems.

School counselors use four primary interventions: *individual and group counseling,* which is confidential and focuses on resolution or constructive coping with problems and concerns; *large-group guidance,* which is planned guidance activities for all students; *consultation,* through collaborative partnership with parents, school, and community personnel on behalf of student success; and *coordination* of school counseling activities. In summary, school counselors hold primary responsibility for developing, implementing, and monitoring the comprehensive school counseling program for their schools. New school counselors, like Zulema, who are familiar with the new vision of school counselors and the ASCA National Model and are well trained in both counseling and leadership skills, enter the professional world of school counseling with the necessary basic preparation. Successful induction into the profession involves the counselor applying what he/she has learned in an environment where there is adequate support and mentoring.

Performance Standards for School Counselors

Like other educational leaders, professional school counselors are expected to be accountable and to meet professional practice standards. Thirteen school counselor performance standards are now included in the accountability section of the ASCA National Model (2003). These basic practice standards for school counselors are summarized in Box 1-1.

This impressive list of performance standards for school counselors implies the need for strong leadership skills. Regardless of the quality of preparation for the profession, school counselors face considerable challenges in their efforts to meet the standards. A foundation of leadership philosophy and perspective provides them with a framework to guide decision making in all aspects of their jobs.

Like many school counselors new to the profession, Zulema was eager to meet and exceed the school counselor performance standards. She sought opportunities to improve the environment in her school for her students and their parents, the teachers, staff, and administrators. Early in her career she was exposed to the ASCA National Model and the Transforming School Counseling Initiative (TSCI), and she was influenced to pursue systemic change in her school. As recommended by ASCA and TSCI, she planned to document the results of her efforts with evidence while applying for Recognized ASCA Model Program (RAMP) status from ASCA.

Zulema's formal counseling and leadership training and development experience during her graduate training program prepared her for effective school counseling and leadership and collaboration in a K–12 setting. Furthermore, Zulema recognized that due to constant changes and challenges in her profession, leadership development is a lifelong process. She decided to continue her formal leadership training beyond completion of her graduate degree. She wished to stay abreast of

---

Box 1-1   School Counselor Performance Standards

---

1. The professional school counselor plans, organizes, and delivers the school counseling program.
2. The professional school counselor implements the school guidance curriculum through the use of effective instructional skills and careful planning of structured group sessions for all students.
3. The professional school counselor implements the individual planning component by guiding individuals and groups of students and their parents through the development of educational and career plans.
4. The professional school counselor provides responsive services through the effective use of individual and small-group counseling, consultation, and referral services.
5. The professional school counselor provides system support through effective school counseling program management and support for other educational programs.
6. The professional school counselor discusses the counseling department management system and the program action plans with the school administrator.
7. The professional school counselor is responsible for establishing and convening an advisory council for the school counseling program.
8. The professional school counselor collects and analyzes data to guide program direction and emphasis.
9. The professional school counselor monitors the students on a regular basis as they progress in school.
10. The professional school counselor uses time and calendar to implement an efficient program.
11. The professional school counselor develops a results evaluation for the program.
12. The professional school counselor conducts a yearly program audit.
13. The professional school counselor is a student advocate, leader, collaborator, and a systems change agent.

From the ASCA National Model, 2003.

---

important developments in her profession and to pursue additional leadership challenges by staying involved in national, state, and local professional school counseling and other educational organizations.

Self-Assessment and Exploration

What do other school personnel expect of school counselors? In order to educate the community and dispel misconceptions about the profession, school counselors today must communicate a clear role definition to administrators, front-desk staff, teachers, parents, school nurses, monitors, and others. To develop an understanding of what others expect of the school counselor in a particular school, it can be helpful to interview them. The following exercise is designed to provide information about how personnel in a particular school perceive the school counseling program and the role of a counselor.

A. Interviews

Instructions: Contact a school administrator (principal or assistant principal), an office staff person, and a school nurse; ask the following questions; and note their responses.

1. What do you view as the most important responsibilities of the school counselor?
2. In what ways do you interact with and/or collaborate with the school counselor in your daily work?
3. What would you like to see the school counselor do that he/she doesn't currently do, or what would you like to see him/her do more of?
4. Rate your understanding of the role of the school counselor on a scale of 1 to 4, where 1 = unclear; 2 = somewhat unclear; 3 = somewhat clear; and 4 = clear. If your rating is lower than 4, what information would help clarify the school counselor's role for you?

Administrator Responses

1. What do you view as the most important responsibilities of the school counselor?

_____

_____

_____

2. In what ways do you interact with and/or collaborate with the school counselor in your daily work?

_____

_____

_____

3. What would you like to see the school counselor do that he/she doesn't currently do, or what would you like to see him/her do more of?

_____

_____

_____

4. Rate your understanding of the role of the school counselor on a scale of 1 to 4, where 1 = unclear; 2 = somewhat unclear; 3 = somewhat clear; and 4 = clear. If your rating is lower than 4, what information would help clarify the school counselor's role for you?

    Circle rating: 1 2 3 4

_____

_____

Office Staff Responses

1. What do you view as the most important responsibilities of the school counselor?

   _____

   _____

   _____

2. In what ways do you interact with and/or collaborate with the school counselor in your daily work?

   _____

   _____

   _____

3. What would you like to see the school counselor do that he/she doesn't currently do, or what would you like to see him/her do more of?

   _____

   _____

   _____

4. Rate your understanding of the role of the school counselor on a scale of 1 to 4, where 1 = unclear; 2 = somewhat unclear; 3 = somewhat clear; and 4 = clear. If your rating is lower than 4, what information would help clarify the school counselor's role for you?

   Circle rating: 1 2 3 4

   _____

   _____

School Nurse Responses

1. What do you view as the most important responsibilities of the school counselor?

   _____

   _____

   _____

2. In what ways do you interact with and/or collaborate with the school counselor in your daily work?

   _____

   _____

   _____

3. What would you like to see the school counselor do that he/she doesn't currently do, or what would you like to see him/her do more of?

_____

_____

_____

4. Rate your understanding of the role of the school counselor on a scale of 1 to 4, where 1 = unclear; 2 = somewhat unclear; 3 = somewhat clear; and 4 = clear. If your rating is lower than 4, what information would help clarify the school counselor's role for you?

Circle rating: 1 2 3 4

_____

_____

B. Sharing Information from the Interviews

When you have obtained responses to these questions, share them with your learning group by posting them as follows:

Instructions: The instructor or facilitator should post four large pieces of paper on the wall (butcher paper works well), one page for each of the questions. Number the sheets at the top by the question and provide a space on each for responses from the three groups. Provide markers for all participants to write their abbreviated responses in the spaces provided. The instructor or facilitator should also post copies of the ASCA description of school counselors' work (Box 1-1) and the Education Trust's new vision of the school counselor (Table 1-1) or make them available for all participants.

C. Discussion

When all responses are noted, discuss as a group the degree to which the responses correspond with the ASCA description of the work of school counselors and the Education Trust's new vision of the school counselor. If there appears to be a lack of alignment, consider as a group what school counselors as educational leaders can do to help align the expectations school personnel have of school counselors with the expectations of ASCA and the Education Trust. If there is alignment, discuss how it may have occurred. In addition, generate further ideas as you continue to read and complete exercises. Make notes of key ideas identified in the discussion.

THE SCHOOL COUNSELOR OF TODAY AND TOMORROW

The current expectations and performance standards for school counselors are clearer than ever, and the bar is set high. School counselors' professional activities are closely tied to the missions of their schools. Yet counselors continue to have hurdles to overcome in most schools in order to achieve optimal effectiveness. These hurdles are typically systems issues in schools, districts, and state departments of education. Examples include: lack of clarity of the school counselor's roles in some schools, unrealistic job expectations, and lack of understanding by teachers and administration of the role of school counselors in achieving the mission of the school. These, as well as other challenges for school counselors in the 21st century, will be explored in depth in Chapter 8.

Many graduate programs in school counseling prepare professional school counselors to practice the "state of the art" school counseling by following the CACREP standards and the practice standards of ASCA. These comprehensive standards ensure quality and consistent preparation of school counseling professionals; however, they cannot anticipate all the unique needs and pressures of particular schools and districts. The unique needs and pressures in a school sometimes create barriers to a school counselor's focus and direction. For example, consider the situation of a recently graduated professional elementary school counselor, Ricardo, at the beginning of his first position in the field.

A NEW SCHOOL COUNSELOR STRUGGLES WITH TEAM PLAYING WHILE ADVOCATING FOR THE PROFESSION

About two months into the first semester of his first counseling position—just after he had developed and was implementing and monitoring the comprehensive school guidance program—Ricardo was unexpectedly assigned by the principal the job of coordination of the standardized testing program for the school. The principal expected him to coordinate the entire school testing program from start to finish, from the initial receipt of test materials to sending out all of the completed tests. This process included tracking all test booklets and ensuring that standardized test procedures were followed.

Case Discussion

Questions About This Case

Before continuing with Ricardo's story, pause to consider the following questions:

- What were the key issues in this scenario that the school counselor as an educational leader needed to consider?
- What were Ricardo's options for responding to the unexpected assignment?
- What are some of the messages the scenario conveys about school counselor roles and priorities?
- How does Ricardo's unexpected assignment align with the new vision of school counselors?
- What can we learn from this scenario about working with the administration in a school?

Further reflection reveals that Ricardo was already stretched to his limit to meet the standards of practice for the profession. Yet he took great pride in being known as a "team player" in the school and, initially, accepted the major assignment without realizing the adverse impact it would have on important portions of the comprehensive school guidance plan. His time and professional expertise were needed to effectively implement, manage, and monitor the guidance plan on a daily basis. Only after accepting the new assignment did Ricardo take some time to reflect and consider the bigger picture. In the process, he realized the compromises required in the school guidance program and his ability to meet student and staff needs if he followed through with the assignment.

After careful consideration, he decided to communicate with the principal, outlining the cost to the comprehensive guidance program and, therefore, the students, if the school counselor took on total responsibility for test coordination. He proposed some options for addressing the issues, including a team effort for coordinating the standardized testing program, and agreed to be part of that team. By being proactive, he hoped to successfully advocate for students, for the school, and for himself as a professional counselor and, at the same time, continue to be a team player.

The principal appreciated Ricardo's assertiveness, his identification of the problem, and the various options he had proposed. He liked the idea of a team approach for the testing program and thanked Ricardo for agreeing to be part of the team. The principal decided to chair the team himself and identified other team members, including a teacher, a librarian, and the school nurse. In retrospect, he had questioned his own decision to ask Ricardo to take on the test coordination and felt relieved that Ricardo approached him about the issue with more viable options. The principal was concerned about not overburdening Ricardo or other school personnel under his leadership.

Further Thoughts on This Case

University training programs can improve the preparation of counselors-in-training for effective leadership by careful placement and supervision in field training that provides students with exposure and coaching in a wide variety of K–12 experiences. Considering scenarios like the one above, counselor educators must present realistic models of school counseling that address rapidly changing demands on schools and school counselors. Graduate programs in school counseling serve students well when they promote counselor leadership skills in school counseling trainees such as clear and assertive communication, effective problem solving, flexibility, adaptability, resilience, creativity, and collaboration within school systems.

In addition to preparing school counseling students for the reality of the changing profession and school environment, counselor educators can advance the profession by actively supporting school counselors and addressing issues that affect them in the field such as the situation Ricardo encountered. They can advocate for them in as many settings as possible: in university training programs, in professional organizations and gatherings, with school administrators, parents, legislators, and the greater community.

Leadership training programs for school counselor trainees are a vehicle that fosters development of leadership skills and characteristics. School counselors become effective educational leaders as they come to recognize the importance of relevant educational leadership concepts such as collaboration, teaming, shared leadership, and a systems perspective. Because of their congruence with basic counseling tenets, these concepts are easily integrated into the counseling preparation curriculum and easily understood and adopted by school counselors. From a big-picture, systems perspective typical of leaders, a school counselor can visualize himself or herself acting as an educational leader, utilizing leadership skills and characteristics to serve as a catalyst for constructive change within school systems. Lao Tzu described the leader's teachers in the following statement (Heider, 1986).

> They moved with grace and awareness, and they were able to negotiate complex situations safely. They were considerate. They did no injury. They were courteous and quiet, like guests. They knew how to yield gracefully and how to be natural and inconspicuous. They were as open and receptive and available as the valleys that lie among the hills.

CHAPTER SUMMARY

School counseling as a profession has only recently developed a clear identity, a national model for school counseling programs, and school counselor performance standards. Early pioneers focused on the vocational guidance role. The greatest progress in clarifying the profession's identity, roles, and standards occurred in the last decade through the efforts of ASCA and the Education Trust. The new-vision model of school counseling developed by the Education Trust and embraced by ASCA views school counselors as educational leaders, advocates, planners, and collaborators.

Recent advances in the school counseling field have greatly benefited school counselors and the K–12 students whom they serve. School counselors who are new to the profession understand their mission and have clear standards to guide their practice. Those entering the profession from graduate training programs in the 21st century are prepared to become effective school leaders who are focused, goal oriented, proactive, and committed to reaching all students. They tend to espouse the philosophy that all children can learn, graduate from high school, and gain access to options for postsecondary training, including college, that leads to satisfying and well-paying jobs. School counselors of the current century and their comprehensive guidance programs are well integrated into the mission of schools.

REVIEW AND REFLECT

1. In small discussion groups, consider the question: Do you believe that all children can learn? What do you see as evidence supporting an affirmative answer? What are some of the reasons given for a negative answer? List the rationale for each response on a large sheet of paper for sharing with the larger group following this small-group activity. Choose someone in your group to summarize the group's responses and rationale for the larger group. Then ask group members to share any changes that may have occurred in their thinking about the initial question.

2. Consider your experience with school counselors in your own K–12 education. List key roles in which you observed them. Then list the key roles that you believe school counselors fill today. Prioritize the top five roles. With a learning partner compare the two lists and discuss similarities and differences between school counselor roles then and now and assess the degree of change you have observed in the profession during your lifetime.

Key Roles of School Counselors in the Past	Key Roles of School Counselors Today
	Circle ranking in top five priorities: None 1 2 3 4 5
	Circle ranking in top five priorities: None 1 2 3 4 5
	Circle ranking in top five priorities: None 1 2 3 4 5
	Circle ranking in top five priorities: None 1 2 3 4 5
	Circle ranking in top five priorities: None 1 2 3 4 5
	Circle ranking in top five priorities: None 1 2 3 4 5
	Circle ranking in top five priorities: None 1 2 3 4 5
	Circle ranking in top five priorities: None 1 2 3 4 5

3. This is another exercise designed to create a perspective of the changes in the school counseling field within the past decade or more. Contact a professional school counselor who has been in the field for at least five years and ask for a brief interview. Ask how long he/she has been in the profession and what major changes have occurred in the field of school counseling over the course of the counselor's service in the profession. Draw a timeline indicating the chronology and estimated time frames of the major changes noted. Bring the timeline to class to share with your group.

RELEVANT WEBSITES

American School Counselor Association: www.schoolcounselor.org
The International Center for Leadership in Education: www.daggett.com/
The School Leadership Development Unit: www.sofweb.vic.edu.au/pd/schlead/
http://21stcenturyschools.northcarolina.edu/center

REFERENCES

American School Counselor Association. (2003). *The ASCA National Model: A framework for school counseling programs.* Alexandria, VA: Author.

American School Counselor Association. (1999). Role statement: The school counselor. *ASCA guide to membership resources.* Alexandria, VA: Author.

Cobia, D. C., & Henderson, D. A. (2003). *Handbook of school counseling.* Upper Saddle River, NJ: Merrill.

Education Trust (1998). *Transforming school counseling initiative* [Brochure]. Denver, CO: The Education Trust.

Gladding, S. T. (1996). *Counseling: A comprehensive profession* (3rd ed.). Upper Saddle River, NJ: Merrill.

Heider, J. (1986). *The tao of leadership.* New York: Bantam Books.

Parsons, F. (1909). *Choosing a vocation.* Boston: Houghton Mifflin.

Rogers, C. (1980). A theory of therapy, personality, and interpersonal relationships as developed in the client-centered framework. In S. Koch (Ed.) *Psychology: A study of science, formulations of the person and the social context* (Vol. 3, pp. 184–256). New York: McGraw-Hill.

Schmidt, John J. (2003). *Counseling in schools: Essential services and comprehensive programs.* Boston: Pearson Education.

Sciarra, D. T. (2004). *School counseling: Foundations and contemporary issues.* Belmont, CA: Brooks/Cole-Thomson Learning.

CHAPTER 2
The Vision: The National Model

A SCHOOL COUNSELING PROGRAM UNDER CONSTRUCTION

Margie was thrilled to be the first full-time school counselor hired for the elementary school where she had been teaching fourth grade for eight years. She had completed her master's degree in school counseling in an evening program at a local university while teaching during the day. Having taught in the school for several years, Margie was familiar with the school culture, including both its resources and its problem areas. She and the other teachers and administrators were concerned about the high rates of tardiness and absenteeism, the low student reading scores on standardized tests, and the family issues that affected many students' ability to learn. A large percentage of the students in the school were of low socioeconomic status, eligible for free and reduced lunches, and were of Hispanic and/or American Indian heritage.

Margie felt her master's degree program in school counseling prepared her well for the challenges she faced in her school. And, while she felt ready for the work before her, she knew it was going to be daunting. She needed to design and implement an elementary school counseling program in her school. The program would need to demonstrate accountability, requiring an evaluation component. Fortunately, Margie would not be alone in the guidance program construction process. She already knew many of the stakeholders who would be eager to assist her as members of the school counseling program advisory council. She also knew many others who would assist her in other, less formal ways. She shared with her school stakeholders a strong sense of the value of the school community and an appreciation of the power inherent in collaborative relationships.

Margie was thankful to be a school counselor in the 21st century. Teachers, administrators, parents, and children have a clearer understanding than ever of the role of school counselors. Additionally, the tools needed to begin her work had recently been developed by the leadership of the ASCA. It was an excellent time to be a school counselor. *The ASCA National Model* had been published in 2003 and the accompanying workbook came out in 2004, giving Margie and her collaborators a framework and tools to move forward in constructing the school's comprehensive counseling program. In Chapter 1 of *The ASCA National Model,* there is a description of a 21st-century school counseling program:

> A school counseling program is comprehensive in scope, preventative in design and developmental in nature. *The ASCA National Model: A Framework for School Counseling Programs* is written to reflect a comprehensive approach to program foundation, delivery system, management system, and accountability. School counseling programs are designed to incorporate proactive school counseling leadership and advocacy to ensure that every student receives the program benefits (ASCA, 2003, p. 13).

Case Discussion

Questions About This Case

- What were some of the opportunities that Margie, as a school counselor leader, identified?
- What tools did she have at her disposal for constructing a comprehensive school counseling program in her school?
- What are some approaches that a school counselor can utilize to engage others in support of the mission of school counselors?
- What messages about school counselor roles and priorities does this scenario convey?
- What can we learn from this case example about working as part of a leadership team in a school?

Further Thoughts on This Case

Margie had a vision of how much better off her students and school would be with the development and implementation of a comprehensive school counseling program. She also had great optimism about the task before her. She had many resources to support her. She was well connected in her school, her district, her community, and her professional organizations. She knew where to begin developing her comprehensive school counseling program and where to obtain the resources, such as a curriculum and potential advisory council members to assist her. She had fostered an outstanding working relationship with her principal; over time, as she progressed in graduate school, she accepted more responsibility as an educational leader. Her principal developed a clear understanding of how school counselors team with administrators and all school personnel to foster student academic success.

Not all school counselors are as fortunate as Margie to have so many resources available. However, other school counselors, regardless of their school atmosphere, can learn from Margie's strengths. She was very good at spotting opportunities among the challenges, and she knew how to take advantage of opportunities that presented themselves. She learned this by becoming aware of her school's needs and keeping her eyes and ears open for the resources that might meet those needs either directly or indirectly. The skills of spotting and taking advantage of opportunities are invaluable leadership and counseling skills that serve school counselors well as they seek to promote the success of their students.

CHAPTER OBJECTIVES

The objectives of this chapter are to:

1. Summarize the National Model for school counseling programs and its implications for school counselor educational leadership.
2. Identify and promote a sense of the common goals of school counselors as educational leaders on a national level within the framework of the National Model.

In Chapter 1, we noted that more than a century of rich history and diverse influences brought the profession of school counseling to the point where it is today. ASCA developed the profession's unified vision and voice in the ASCA National Model (ASCA, 2003), briefly summarized here.

ASCA (1998) described the purpose of the school counseling program as "to affect specific skills and learning opportunities through academic, career, and personal/social development experiences in a proactive and preventive manner for all students." The primary goal of school counseling programs is to promote and enhance student learning through the three areas listed above. School counseling leadership and advocacy efforts within the counseling program have an impact on student developmental progress from prekindergarten through high school and beyond. In 1998, ASCA developed national standards for K–12 students who have school counseling programs in their schools. There are three standards in each of three areas of student development: academic, career, and personal/social. Each standard includes expected student competencies, and the competencies include desired student outcomes. The school counselor as educational leader develops and implements the school counseling program to ensure that all students meet the competencies.

The ASCA National Model was presented to the professional organization in 2003 as a blueprint for designing and implementing an effective school counseling program. Starting at the ASCA national convention in June 2004, with similar plans for the following conventions, ASCA acknowledged several schools as RAMPs for having documented evidence that they had followed the model. The National Model offers a detailed outline for a comprehensive approach to school counseling programs that requires strong school counselor leadership, including program foundation, delivery system, management system, and accountability (ASCA, 2003). The model incorporates the ASCA National Standards (1998) for student development promoting academic success for all students. A workbook has been published (2004) to guide school counselor leaders in aligning their programs with the National Model.

In addition to being comprehensive, the ASCA National Model is preventive, developmental, and designed to support the academic mission of the school. The school counselor's role is to be an educational leader and agent of systemic change. ASCA advocates implementation of the model by professional school counselors with at least master's degrees who have credentials in their states.

Shortly after the National Model was published and distributed, schools across the nation began to implement it. Some schools chose to apply to become RAMP-designated schools. The school counselors in those schools took responsibility for documenting the alignment of their school counseling programs with the National Model. In addition, the counselors completed application forms and submitted them to ASCA for review by a committee that determined whether the program met RAMP criteria.

Self-Assessment and Exploration

In this exercise, you will review the actual RAMP application and interview the counselor at a school that has RAMP designation.

1. Visit the ASCA website at www.schoolcounselor.org, find the link for the RAMP application, and either review it online or download it and review it.
2. Based on your experience with school counseling programs, identify the areas in which it would be easiest to align a school counseling program with the National Model and the areas that might be difficult to align.

Areas that are easy to align:

_____

_____

_____

_____

_____

_____

_____

Areas that are difficult to align:

_____

_____

_____

_____

_____

_____

What makes some areas easier to align and others more difficult?

_____

_____

_____

_____

_____

_____

_____

3. Do you know of a school counseling program that has RAMP designation? If yes, contact the counselor at that school and ask about the process involved to apply for and receive RAMP designation. If no, try contacting a RAMP school listed on the ASCA RAMP website.
4. Ask the counselor at the RAMP school if ensuring that the school counseling program was aligned with the National Model made a difference in the school and, if so, what difference it made.

_____

_____

_____

_____

_____

ELEMENTS OF THE ASCA NATIONAL MODEL

The ASCA National Model consists of four elements: program foundation, delivery system, management system, and accountability.

Program Foundation

The foundation element focuses on four areas related to setting the stage for what students need to know and what they need to be able to do. A school counseling program should be built around a set of principles or a philosophy agreed upon by the leaders and advisers for the school. The National Model recommends a process for developing a list of assumptions of an agreed-upon philosophy. It suggests that all counseling team members first examine their own personal beliefs as they answer the following seven questions (ASCA, 2003). Self-examination is an important process in the ongoing development of counselors and other educational leaders. The model encourages the counseling team to then come together as a group and develop consensus regarding the statement of philosophy for the team's program.

1. What do we believe about achievement for every student?
2. Do we believe all students can achieve, given proper support?

3. Do we believe there are differences in learning styles for students and that children respond differently? How do we react to those responses?
4. What do we believe about the program's ability to provide academic, career, and personal/social development for every student?
5. When we look at the school's mission of academic achievement, what responsibility does the school counseling program have to support this mission?
6. What do we believe about educational reform and the school counselor's role in it?
7. What do we believe about the role of parents or guardians, staff, and community members within the school counseling program?

The National Model provides some guidelines for philosophy statements that are recommended as a minimum for adoption by every school. These guidelines include a focus on all students, a statement about the ability of all students to achieve, and the use of data to drive program decisions. Components of the philosophy statements can be composed from the ideas that are generated from the responses to the seven questions above.

In addition to an agreed-upon philosophy, the school counseling program's architects should continue in their roles as educational leaders by developing a clear mission statement with a purpose and vision relevant to every student in the school. The school counseling program's mission statement should be designed to be consistent by linking to the general educational mission statements of the school, the district, the state department of education, and ultimately, the U.S. Department of Education. In addition, the school counseling program's mission statement should align with the mission statements of the school district's school counseling department, the state's school counseling professional organization, and the ASCA National Model.

The ASCA National Standards and competencies (Campbell & Dahir, 1997) identify expected student knowledge, attitudes, and skills in the three domains of academic, career, and personal/social development. These standards and competencies represent the desired results of an effective school counseling program. School counselors as educational leaders are held accountable for demonstrating outcomes related to their programs. They demonstrate accountability by collecting data and reporting evidence of students meeting the standards and competencies.

Self-Assessment and Exploration

In this exercise, you will use the seven questions regarding a philosophy statement found at the beginning of this section. You are expected to act as educational leaders as you work within a small group to develop consensus on a statement of philosophy for a school counseling program.

Instructions: Divide into small learning groups and imagine that group members are all counselors in the same school. Designate someone from each group to take notes on a large sheet of paper.

1. Discuss and agree on an answer to each of the seven questions, and post it on the wall.

2. On a separate piece of large paper, write a concise statement of philosophy based on the answers to those questions.

3. Join together again in the large group and share the small groups' philosophy statements.

4. Develop a statement of philosophy for the large group based on common themes from the smaller groups.

5. Comment on your observations of what you viewed as leadership behaviors within your small and large groups.

Delivery System

The National Model delivery system has four components: the school guidance curriculum; the individual student plan; services responsive to the immediate needs of students; and system support activities, such as committee involvement, program management, and professional development. The school counselor as educational leader is expected to collaborate with a wide variety of school and community members who have an impact on students' lives, including but not limited to: school administrators, parents/guardians, teachers, school psychologists, school nurses, school social workers, and school resource officers. Within the delivery system, the school counselor must wear many hats with corresponding leadership activities such as program development and planning, consulting and coaching, proactively responding to immediate student needs, teaming and collaborating, managing, and training.

School Guidance Curriculum

The school guidance curriculum consists of the written school counseling lessons that are delivered to all students. The school counselor takes leadership responsibility for the curriculum's design, implementation, and evaluation. The curriculum is the vehicle for transferring the knowledge and skills deemed necessary by ASCA for all students to achieve success in the three domains of academic achievement, career development, and personal/social growth. Counselors can deliver the curriculum through various means, including classroom instruction, integration of curriculum with academic subject matter, small-group activities outside the classroom, and workshops for parents.

Individual Student Planning

School counselors as school leaders are responsible for coordinating individual student planning and student evaluation of educational, occupational, and personal goals. They are proactive in assisting students with transitions. They provide individual planning services through one-on-one meetings or small groups in which they may administer interest inventories; review, analyze, and interpret test scores; provide information on promotion and retention; facilitate career exploration and decisions; review behavior plans; and so on.

Responsive Services

Responsive services are designed to meet the immediate needs of students through the provision of information, counseling, consultation, peer facilitation, and referral. These services fall on a continuum with early intervention at one end and crisis intervention at the other end. The school counselor as educational leader is often the first-line contact and has a major role in determining which services are most appropriate for students in immediate need.

System Support

School counselors provide system support by accepting leadership and management responsibility for establishing, maintaining, and continuously improving the school counseling program. They attend and provide ongoing professional development activities. They consult, as necessary, with members of the larger school system. They partner, collaborate, and team with colleagues in the interest of supporting the local, state, and national missions of the public educational system.

Management System

The management system for school counseling programs consists of the clearly defined processes and tools necessary to effectively manage a school counseling program, including management agreements, an advisory council, data, action plans, and the use of time and calendars. Management agreements are statements of expectations for individual school counselors negotiated by counselors and their administrators. The agreements include expected program responsibilities and student outcomes. They document school counselors' accountability for their programs.

The advisory council reviews, advises, and assists the school counseling program within a district. It should include a broad representation of stakeholders, including counselors, students, parents, teachers, administrators, and community members. It serves as a mechanism for review and recommendations from various stakeholders of the school.

The school counselor leader uses data to assess the needs of students and to guide the development of school counseling programs. The school counselor also uses data to demonstrate the level of effectiveness of counseling interventions. Outcome data provides important feedback for future planning of school counseling programs. School counseling programs with evidence of their effectiveness can be shared with other professional school counselors who, in turn, can implement similar programs.

The school counselor uses the leadership skills of developing, planning, and organizing to create or locate and implement an appropriate guidance curriculum. The National Model describes guidance curriculum action plans and closing-the-gap action plans. A description of each of these action plans follows. The two work hand in hand. The *guidance curriculum action plan* addresses domains, standards, and competencies from the ASCA National Standards (Campbell & Dahir, 1997). Domain refers to the broad developmental area to be addressed. The ASCA National Standards include three domains: academic, career, and personal/social. Standards refer to statements describing what students are expected to know and be able to do within a certain domain. There are a total of nine national standards, three in each of the three domains. Competencies refer to specific expectations of student achievement in a content standard area. The ASCA National Standards include a total of 122 competencies for students. Here is an example from the ASCA National Standards:

Domain: Academic

Standard A: Students will acquire the attitudes, knowledge, and skills that contribute to effective learning in school and across the life span

Competency A: A2.0: Acquire skills for improving learning.

In addition to components of the ASCA National Standards, the guidance curriculum action plan includes a description of guidance lessons, materials, a timeline for completion, the person responsible for delivery, and methods of evaluating student success. The school counselor educational leader uses the closing-the-gap action plan to address gaps between current educational data for the school and desired results. For optimal effectiveness as an educational leader who documents and shares data regarding progress in closing the gap, the school counselor must become familiar with and committed to the use of data for planning and goal setting.

The National Model guidelines call for school counselors to spend the largest portion of their time providing direct services to students. Counselors provide prevention and intervention services. They use their leadership planning and organization skills in implementing their management system through planning the timeline for service delivery. They develop a master calendar and weekly, monthly, and annual calendars that outline implementation of the school guidance program guided by the management agreement, advisory council recommendations, guidance curriculum, and closing-the-gap action plans. To keep stakeholders informed about the school counseling program and to demonstrate school counselor accountability, the school counselor uses leadership skills of communication by publishing and making the school calendars available for review.

Accountability

The National Model is results oriented, indicating the need for the school counselor leader to begin planning the school guidance program with current data, clear goals in mind, and collection of outcome data that is shared with stakeholders and analyzed for program improvement efforts. It includes performance standards for school counselors that relate directly to the development, planning, and implementation of the school counseling program.

A program audit is built into the National Model to assist school counselors and other stakeholders in ensuring that their school counseling program aligns with the ASCA National Model. The audit can determine areas for clarification and improvement. The school counselor uses the leadership skill of incorporating feedback into the school counseling program on a continuous basis, making adjustments to constantly improve it.

THEMES OF THE ASCA NATIONAL MODEL

The National Model embraces the themes of the Education Trust's (1997) National Initiative for Transforming School Counseling: leadership, advocacy, collaboration and teaming, and systemic change. In the transformed, or new-vision, role, school counselors are expected to accept leadership roles within their schools, districts, professional organizations, and beyond to promote the goal of high-quality education for all students and equal access to higher education.

School counselors as leaders are called upon to be advocates for the academic success of all students. This translates into developing strategies for removing barriers to student success. Often, the school counselor collaborates with internal and external stakeholders to accomplish systemic change. School counselors have a unique knowledge base and training experience that makes them well qualified to develop and maintain effective working relationships with school stakeholders. Formal training in leadership skills offers them additional tools to effectively carry out their mission. Data collection and analysis are leadership activities critical to removing barriers to student success. School counselors must be prepared to work with school data on an ongoing basis. They need to gain access to and become familiar with their school's data regarding student placement, student academic achievement, attendance, course-enrollment patterns, drop-out rates, and so on. These data offer insights for school counselors and other educational leaders regarding areas to target for systemic change.

CHAPTER SUMMARY

The ASCA National Model offers a framework for comprehensive school guidance programs as well as guidelines for school counselor leadership activities. With knowledge of the National Standards for student competencies and the ASCA National Model for school counseling programs, the wise recommendations of a diverse and representative advisory council, and by teaming with the school's administrative leadership, a school counselor can effectively design, implement, and evaluate a school counseling program. Furthermore, as school counselors across the country align with this national framework, the vision of school counselors as educational leaders addressing the academic, personal, and career needs of all students can become a reality.

REVIEW AND REFLECT

1. Gather and compare several organizational mission statements. Choose statements from a school guidance program, the district's guidance department, the state's school counseling professional organization, the ASCA, and the U.S. Department of Education.
2. Identify areas of consistency or discrepancy among the documents.
3. In what ways can the mission statements be more closely aligned?

RELEVANT WEBSITES

American School Counselor Association: www.schoolcounselor.org
The Education Trust: www.edtrust.org

REFERENCES

American School Counselor Association. (2003). *The ASCA national model: A framework for school counseling programs.* Alexandria, VA: Author.

American School Counselor Association (1998). *The national standards for school counseling programs.* Alexandria, VA: American School Counselor Association.

Campbell, C. A., & Dahir, C. (1997). *Sharing the vision: The national standards for school counseling programs.* Alexandria, VA: Authors.

Education Trust. (1997). *The national guidance and counseling reform program.* Washington, DC: Author.

CHAPTER 3

The Mandate for School Counselor Leadership

A SCHOOL COUNSELOR CALLED TO LEAD

Carrie began her career as a school counselor following four successful years teaching English to high school freshmen. During her last two and a half years as a teacher, she taught during the day and worked on her master's degree in school counseling in the evenings. She had a passion for helping students and encouraging them to achieve their academic potential. When she began her work as a secondary school counselor, she expected to be called upon to serve in some leadership roles not required of her as a teacher. She enthusiastically accepted the role of school representative on a district-wide crisis intervention team and on the counselor professional development team. Carrie also served as editor of the state school counselor newsletter. She was comfortable in these roles, and her contributions were valued and appreciated. She developed a reputation as a hard worker and a team player who made significant contributions in planning the comprehensive guidance program in her school and who promptly followed through with committee assignments.

In her second year as a high school counselor, her counseling department chair retired rather suddenly and earlier than expected due to a combination of health and personal problems. The other two counselors in the department were planning to retire within the next one or two years and were not interested in the position. Her principal strongly encouraged Carrie to apply for the counseling department chair position because she had been so successful as a teacher, school counselor, and committee member. Carrie felt ambivalent. On the one hand, she was flattered by the principal's encouragement, and she wanted the challenge of the position. She believed she could make a significant difference at a systemic level if she was effective in this leadership position. While in graduate school, she had become familiar with and committed to the changes proposed in the roles of school counselors by the Transforming School Counseling Initiative of the Education Trust (1998). She also felt a strong commitment to the ASCA National Model (2003) and had a desire to implement a comprehensive school counseling program based on the national model.

On the other hand, she felt ill prepared for this leadership opportunity and lacked confidence in her leadership abilities. She worried that because she had limited experience and was the newest and youngest member of her department, she might have little credibility as a leader. She feared the resistance of her counseling colleagues, who had indicated that they were not interested in leadership or other changes in their roles during their limited remaining tenure. Carrie had no sense of where to begin to address the gaps in her leadership development in order to be effective in her school environment.

Case Discussion

Questions About This Case

- What were some of the key issues that this school counselor needed to consider in making her decision about whether to accept a leadership position?
- What other options did she have in responding to the opportunity to accept a formal leadership position in her school?
- What are some ways a school counselor can prepare to become a leader?
- What messages about school counselor roles and priorities does this scenario convey?
- What can we learn from this case example about working with administrators and other school counselors in a school?

Further Thoughts on This Case

Carrie sought the advice of two of her mentors. She spoke to her adviser from graduate school, who helped her explore some of her options. For example, Carrie could choose not to apply for the position and continue her leadership development at her own pace. She could apply for the position and if it were offered to her, negotiate for leadership coaching services for the first year. Or, she could apply for the position and if it were offered to her, enroll in a formal leadership training program through her district or the university.

The other mentor from whom she sought advice was a guidance department chair at another high school who had supervised Carrie's internship experience. He shared his belief that she had strong leadership potential and predicted a high likelihood of success if she were placed in the department chair position. He also gave Carrie an overview of his duties and described what he liked and disliked about his position, what he found most rewarding, and what he found most challenging. He agreed to continue to mentor Carrie if she were chosen as the department chair at her school and offered to meet with her on a regular basis at least during her first year in the job.

After consulting with her mentors, Carrie decided to apply for the position, and shortly after interviewing for it, she was offered the position. She accepted after negotiating for time off to attend a formal leadership training program at the local university, paid for by her school district. She felt supported by her principal and her district and looked forward to a rewarding collaborative relationship with her principal and a challenging new position that would keep her motivated to learn all that she could to be a more effective educational leader.

CHAPTER OBJECTIVES

The objectives of this chapter are to:

1. Explore the mandate for school counselor leadership.
2. Identify key areas for systemic change in K–12 schools.

The information in this chapter provides background and support for the material in the following chapters which will address challenges ahead, educational leadership theory, personal leadership assessment, review of assessment results, planning for leadership improvement, following an advocacy model, effective collaboration, and understanding and aligning the school counseling program with the National Model using a data-driven approach.

MEETING PERFORMANCE STANDARDS

An examination of current expectations of school counselors makes a strong case for school counselor leadership. For example, a review of the 13 ASCA performance standards for school counselors (listed in Chapter 1) suggests that leadership skills are necessary for success in meeting the standards. The performance standards include leadership activities such as planning, organizing, consultation, program management, establishing and convening an advisory council, collecting and analyzing data to guide program direction and emphasis, evaluating results, conducting an annual program audit, and infusing themes of student advocacy, educational reform, equity, community, teaming, and systems change into the school environment. Counselors are expected to coordinate all aspects of their school counseling programs. They are involved in system-wide planning, developing K–12 guidance curriculum and doing individual planning for students. They provide responsive services such as individual and group counseling, crisis counseling, and consultation. They provide system support for setting goals, assisting in research and development, and conducting activities related to staff and community public relations. They participate on and chair school and district committees. School counselors who lack at least some basic leadership training and development are at a disadvantage.

FACING CHALLENGING SOCIAL ISSUES

In addition to the demands of the school system, school counselors are challenged by current social issues in the larger society. Economic concerns, the high rate of divorce, the number of single parents, welfare reforms, and increasing violence and safety issues in our schools are just a few circumstances that commonly affect families and children. These factors suggest the need for counselors to be proactive as leaders and advocates. In these roles, counselors can empower both themselves and others to "collaborate in the service of shared visions, values, and missions" (Bolman & Deal, 1994).

Social justice leadership and advocacy require counselor actions to ensure that all students have equal access to opportunities and services that enhance their positions in life. According to Lee and Walz (1998), social action is based on two premises: that the environment affects behavior and that counselors are socially, morally, and professionally responsible for addressing social issues. Every client, regardless of race, culture, ethnicity, religious orientation, or socioeconomic status is entitled to equal access to opportunity. School counselors are in an excellent position to direct their own behaviors toward the goal of eliminating environmental obstacles to social justice for their students. Bradley and Lewis (2000) maintained that all counselors can play a more active part in addressing societal issues.

Menacker (1976) pointed out that counselors may identify harmful institutional policies and take action to change them. Advocacy counseling typically requires the school counselor as leader to take risks on behalf of students. Yet in schools, like other institutions, diplomacy can minimize negative responses from teachers and administrators (Ponzo, 1974). Leadership and advocacy counseling in schools requires school counselors to become familiar with potential resources. The school counselor/social advocate must be creative and skilled in identifying allies and enlisting their support for the cause in focus. Furthermore, school counselor leaders must be assertive to be most effective in the role of advocate for all students.

Assertiveness is a skill that one can learn and develop. It refers to openly expressing one's expectations, opinions, beliefs, and feelings while respecting others. It is not the same as being aggressive, which refers to expressing oneself in an abrasive manner. It is also different than being passive, which refers to suppressing one's ideas. The following assertiveness exercise is provided to help you to assess your own level of assertiveness.

Self-Assessment and Exploration

In this set of exercises, you will assess your own assertiveness and compare your assessment with others who will rate you.

A. Rate Yourself on an Assertiveness Scale

Instructions: Based on the situations stated in the items that follow, rate how assertive you believe you would be in a school setting, using the 1–10 scale provided, where 1 is extremely passive, and 10 is exceptionally assertive.

1. Criticizing a colleague

   1   2   3   4   5   6   7   8   9   10

2. Expressing anger toward a colleague

   1   2   3   4   5   6   7   8   9   10

3. Speaking out publicly about an important issue

   1   2   3   4   5   6   7   8   9   10

4. Persisting and not being worn down in a fight for rights

   1   2   3   4   5   6   7   8   9   10

5. Expressing one's full range of feelings around colleagues

   1   2   3   4   5   6   7   8   9   10

6. Insisting that others correct their mistakes

   1   2   3   4   5   6   7   8   9   10

7. Speaking up at meetings

   1   2   3   4   5   6   7   8   9   10

8. Insisting that others do their fair share on a project

   1   2   3   4   5   6   7   8   9   10

9. Showing love and affection for those with whom one works

   1   2   3   4   5   6   7   8   9   10

10. Publicly accepting responsibility for making a mistake

   1   2   3   4   5   6   7   8   9   10

Scoring: Maximum score equals 100.

Assertive:	70–100
Somewhat Assertive:	50–69
Unassertive:	1–49

Consider your overall score to get a sense of how assertive you are. Then look at the individual items to determine if there are particular situations that pose difficulty for you. You might incorporate these in your leadership improvement plan to be developed in an exercise in a later chapter.

B. Ask a Colleague to Rate You

Have a colleague who knows you fairly well rate you using this scale and then compare your rating with your colleague's rating. Discuss any large gaps between the ratings. In their text on school counseling, Baker and Gerler (2004) noted, "…School counseling is a human service career, and school counselors are exposed to numerous situations that challenge their ability to serve all clients who are in need. We believe that leadership and collaboration are avenues through which school counselors can be of greater service to a broad range of clients. Perhaps the most important ingredients are the desire and will to do so" (p. 318).

Effective leadership is critical to assertive response and advocacy for student needs. Although the demands on school counselors to be leaders and advocates are greater than ever, school counselor education programs have only recently begun to significantly address these demands. School counselor education programs typically do not include training specifically focused on assertive leadership and advocacy. School counselors need to be adequately prepared to meet the expectations placed on them when they enter the K–12 work setting. Resources are readily available in the great body of literature that exists on educational leadership. This material is easily integrated into the graduate school counseling curriculum to provide trainees with the necessary knowledge and skills.

THE WATERFALL STORY

Many practicing school counselors have heard the story of "the babies and the waterfall," frequently told by Pat Martin when she was a senior specialist at the Education Trust focusing her efforts on the Transforming School Counseling Initiative. The story is a metaphor for the process of transforming school counseling. As the authors remember, it went something like this:

Early in Pat's career as a school counselor, she likened her work to standing at the bottom of a waterfall over which many babies were falling. They were falling all over the place in the pool below the waterfall, to the right and left of her, in front of and behind her. Pat imagined herself doing her best to catch as many of the babies as possible, and she sincerely wanted to save every one of them. She worked very hard at saving babies. But there were so many babies falling that she could not keep up with the need.

It was not long before Pat realized that she could catch only so many babies. She was losing many babies, and she was exhausted from saving the few she could catch. Pat did not give up, but she realized that she needed to approach the problem from a different perspective. She decided to devote her efforts to organizing a group of concerned individuals and leading them to the top of the waterfall where they would construct a safety net that would prevent the babies from falling over in the first place.

Many school counselors strongly relate to this story. They feel passion for their work and have a commitment to the children and families they serve. They also experience the exhaustion and futility of trying to save one child at a time when so many need attention. Nevertheless, some school counselors believe it is their noble calling to "catch the babies at the bottom of the waterfall." They work hard to make a difference in the lives of the children they encounter and are appreciated for what they do. Meanwhile, however, all around them, other children who have not come to their attention or who must wait for an intervention may be losing ground in their struggle to succeed personally, academically, and practically. In the text *The Professional School Counselor*, Studer (2005) expands on the issue of school counselors who continue to work under the traditional model.

Many practicing school counselors trained under this traditional model continue "business as usual" and are reluctant to embrace a comprehensive developmental approach to counseling. Although these counselors are well-guided in their belief that what they are currently doing is working—and in many cases *is* working, they have rarely taken the time to evaluate their effectiveness. The future school counselor will receive training and support in organizational skills, knowledge of the new model, and confidence to advocate for this approach to counseling program delivery (p. 24).

Fortunately, not only the newly trained school counselors, but also a growing number of traditionally trained school counselors have realized, like Pat Martin, that the only way to save the babies is to lead and to advocate for systems change, which would, in essence, put a net across the top of the waterfall and keep the babies from falling. In a major step toward that goal, Martin accepted a leadership role with the Education Trust, an independent nonprofit organization supported by the Dewitt Wallace-Reader's Digest Fund, to transform the school counseling profession. The following is its mission statement:

> The Education Trust works for the high academic achievement of all students at all levels, kindergarten through college, and forever closing the achievement gaps that separate low-income students and students of color from other students. Our basic tenet is this—All children will learn at high levels when they are taught to high levels.

TRANSFORMING SCHOOL COUNSELING

Starting in the mid 1990s, Pat Martin, her colleague Reese House, and others from the Education Trust worked closely with six universities that received large grants from the Education Trust to research what changes were needed to improve school counseling effectiveness and how to go about transforming the profession, including school counseling preparation programs, to align with identified needed improvements. Martin, House, and others at the Education Trust are well known as visionaries and advocates currently in the field of school counseling. They have led the way for school counselors as leaders, advocates, collaborators, and catalysts for systemic change.

The Education Trust's research (1997) identified and addressed eight essential elements for substantive systems change to make school counseling education programs more effective. Table 3-1 includes the elements identified as targets for change.

Each of the eight elements for change in Table 3-1 is accompanied by a brief explanation of guidelines for the transformation of existing university school counseling programs. The overarching objective was a substantial change in the philosophy and mission of school counseling programs as well as the manner in which school counseling programs were delivered and the use and expectations of school counselors who were prepared by transformed university programs. Today, transformed graduate school counseling programs are aligned with and support the current ASCA mission for school counselors: to provide services to *all students* to promote academic success and access to postsecondary education.

The main thrust of the recommended changes was to prepare new school counselors for the demands of twenty-first century schools and to foster a new vision of school counselors as leaders, advocates for systems change and social justice, and collaborators on behalf of all students. The Education Trust and the American School Counselor Association have also made concerted efforts to effect change in the way

Table 3-1   Eight Essential Elements for Systems Change in Schools/Counseling Preparation Programs

Essential Elements	Explanation of Elements
1. Criteria for selection and recruitment of candidates for counselor preparation programs	School counseling recruitment should focus on attracting and selecting students from diverse backgrounds interested in developing leadership, advocacy, and collaboration skills designed to meet the academic needs of all students.
2. Curricular content, structure, and sequence of courses	Curriculum should emphasize knowledge and skills of academic and career guidance for all students rather than personal or college counseling for only a few students. Curriculum should address current roles of counselors and include exposure to the ASCA National Model and the ASCA National Standards.
3. Methods of instruction, field experiences and practices	Integration of university and field training experiences starting early in the program and emphasizing practice of what is learned in the classroom. Field-based approaches in school settings working with diverse student populations are recommended.
4. Induction process into the profession	Ongoing supervised experiences in the school setting and mentoring that starts in graduate school and continues during transition into the school counseling profession and beyond. This involves collaborative efforts between K–12 and higher education institutions.
5. Working relationships with community partners	Emphasis on the intentional coordinated development of relationships between students and staff from community resources that provide opportunities for learning about diverse cultures and their needs.
6. Professional development activities of counselor educators	Counselor educators within a program need to plan their own professional development to foster shared understanding of the stated philosophy and values for the program and to address student and institutional needs as identified by data.
7. University/school system partnerships	School districts, universities, and state departments of education should partner and work toward agreement about graduate training programs, credentialing, and school district requirements for school counselors.
8. University/state department partnerships	Universities should be involved in working relationships with the state department of education efforts regarding changes in K–12 guidance credentialing requirements and in conducting and providing research to guide program revisions.

counselors in the field were doing business. Both organizations viewed school counselors as ideally positioned to advocate for students as educational leaders in K–12 reform. Prior to the transforming school counseling initiative, school counselors had been left out of K–12 reform efforts.

Commonly Identified Areas for Change Efforts in Schools

Data from the U.S. Census Bureau (March, 2000) indicate that students in this country graduate at different rates. By age 24, 94 percent of Asian students, 91 percent of white students, 87 percent of African American students, and only 62 percent of Latino students graduate from high school. Public schools in the United

Table 3-2   17-Year-Olds' Reading Skills

	African American	Latino American	European American
Learn from specialized materials	1%	2%	8%
Understand complicated information	17%	24%	46%
Make generalizations	95%	97%	98%

Data from National Center for Educational Statistics, 1999.

Table 3-3   17-Year-Olds' Math Skills

	African American	Latino American	European American
Multistep problem solving	1%	3%	10%
Moderately complex procedures	27%	38%	70%
Numerical operations	89%	94%	99%

Data from National Center for Educational Statistics, 1999.

States are not graduating all students. In addition, the population of students in U.S. schools today is very different from the population of yesterday.

The same U.S. Census Bureau data also tell us that low-income students attend postsecondary institutions at lower rates than high-income students. No Child Left Behind (NCLB) legislation was designed to address these gaps in achievement.

Additional data from the National Center for Educational Statistics (1999) indicate that too few 17-year-olds demonstrate strong reading and math skills. These data are summarized in Tables 3-2 and 3-3.

The transformed school counseling profession has aligned its mission and its activities with the mission of schools. School counselors, like teachers, administrators, and other educational staff are concerned with the academic success of all students and with closing achievement gaps among students. School counselors have joined the educational reform efforts of the schools and are emerging leaders in these efforts. Using national, state, and local educational data in support of the mission of schools is critical to the activities of school counselors.

New jobs in the workforce are requiring greater education than in the past (Fleetwood & Shelley, 2000; Braddock, 1999).

- 70 percent of the thirty fastest-growing jobs will require an education beyond high school.
- 40 percent of all new jobs will require at least an associate's degree.
- The total number of college-level job openings between 1990 and 2008 will nearly equal the number of college-educated entrants to the workforce.

Table 3-4   Measure of Academic Progress (MAP) in Three Public School Third Grades in Douglas, Arizona (OYG = one year of growth)

School	OYG Math	OYG Reading
A Avenue Elementary School	77%	35%
Clawson School	65%	43%
Faras School	76%	38%

Data from Arizona Department of Education, September 20, 2004.

Table 3-5   Measure of Academic Progress (MAP) in Three Charter School Third Grades in Tucson, Arizona (OYG = one year of growth)

School	OYG Math	OYG Reading
Academy of Tucson	67%	87%
Accelerated Learning Lab	86%	75%
Carden School of Tucson	58%	45%

Data from Arizona Department of Education, September 20, 2004.

The Need for Relevant Guidance

If students are to be successful academically and in their careers, school counselors must provide guidance so that students understand workforce demands, their post-secondary-school options, and how to adequately prepare for their chosen careers. In order to provide relevant guidance, school counselors need to be familiar with current data regarding national and local workforce trends and requirements.

In addition to staying abreast of national data, school counselor educational leaders need to be aware of trends in their states, districts, and their own buildings. These data are readily available. For instance, the Arizona Department of Education releases a Measure of Academic Progress (MAP) annually. These data are available from the state department of education and are also published in local newspapers. Students in each school are tracked for the most recent two school years to determine if one year of growth (OYG) was made in the second year based on Stanford achievement test scores. The emphasis is on progress from the prior year. Table 3-4 shows a sample data table for three public school third grades in Douglas, Arizona. Table 3-5 shows a sample data table for three charter school third grades in Tucson, Arizona.

SCHOOL COUNSELORS USE THEIR COLLECTIVE VOICE

It is also useful for school counselors as leaders in education to be aware of trends in their profession at various levels and to seek opportunities to let their voices be heard about progress and issues in the field. For instance, by participating in surveys regarding the profession, they can help create data that can lead to change when it is

Table 3-6   Areas of School-Related Counselor Concerns Reported on Arizona School Counselor Survey, 2004

	Elementary School	Middle School	High School
Areas of concern (in order based on number of counselors marking the concern)	Academic issues	Academic issues	Academic issues
	Family/home issues	Study skills	Family/home issues
	Grief/loss	Family/home issues	Depression
	Hyperactivity	Time management	Achievement testing
	Attention deficit	Grief and loss issues	Grief and loss issues
	Peer conflicts	Hyperactivity	Hyperactivity
	Anger	Attention deficit	Attention deficit
	Social skills	Peer conflicts	Relationship issues
	Self-image	Anger	Time management
	Abuse by parents	Social skills	Scheduling
	Food/clothing needs	Teacher conflicts	Disciplinary issues
	Shyness	Career exploration	Peer conflicts
		Depression	Study skills
		Relationship issues	Self-image
		Racism/prejudice	Anger management
		Anxiety	Scholarships/college
			College preparation
			Home concerns
			Teacher conflicts
			Disability issues
			English language
			Career issues
			Anxiety
			Food/clothing needs

Kolodinsky, DeVoss, Brown, Montopoli, & Moore, 2004.

presented to the educational community. A recent unpublished survey of 120 Arizona school counselors (Kolodinsky, DeVoss, Brown, Montopoli, & Moore, 2004) was designed to assess job satisfaction, areas of frustration, breadth of day-to-day activities, comfort/competency in working with various psychosocial issues in today's schools, degree of alignment with comprehensive competency-based guidance, city-to-city and level-to-level comparisons, and types of professional development training sought. The results helped the researchers speculate about current concerns of school counselors in Arizona.

Table 3-6 summarizes the areas of concern of Arizona school counselors for their students by elementary, middle-, and high school level. These areas of concern offer a starting point for identifying targets for systems change. The counselors and other stakeholders could follow up by exploring existing data or collecting new data to determine the extent of the problem in a district or in specific schools. The data can enlighten and guide the group in decision making about what issues need to be addressed on a school- or district-wide change agenda.

Areas of professional training sought by the school counselors in the Arizona survey reflected the counselors' concerns about issues facing students. The training was needed in areas including understanding medical diagnoses and needs, helping English-language learners, immigration issues, eating disorders, gang involvement, rape counseling and sexual abuse, anger management, adolescent counseling, suicide, and depression. The top three areas of need for professional training for counselors in the same Arizona survey were anger management, adolescent counseling, and child and adolescent depression.

School counselor frustrations enumerated in this study were: feeling overwhelmed with duties, having to do meaningless tasks, wasting time with new data systems, credit checks, scheduling, not being able to do classroom guidance, getting pulled into the classroom as a teacher, which takes away from counselor duties, too many other job pressures taking away from counseling, high parental expectation of schools but low parental involvement, and too many other duties during noncontract hours.

The school counselors in the study were also concerned that some children get little support or opportunity at home for growth. It is difficult not to be able to change children's home lives and to cope with parental apathy. Counselors reported feeling challenged when working with parents who deny their child's problem, whether it is depression, bullying, or lack of follow-through. School counselors are limited in what they can do when they make a referral for a student and the parents do not utilize the recommended outside services..

The areas of concern for students displayed in Table 3-6, the areas of professional training sought and the frustrations encountered by the counselors who responded to the Arizona survey indicate issues to examine more closely with either existing data or a plan to collect new data. The data will point to areas for targeting systems change efforts within the school system.

Identifying Targets for Change

The purpose of this exercise is to stimulate reflection on some of the existing problems in schools and/or districts that might be targeted for change by a school leadership team.

1. Identify one problem in a local school or district for which you would like to see the school counselor involved as a leader of systemic change efforts.
2. Where do you think you might find data to assist in substantiating this problem in the school or district?
3. Who would be the key stakeholders for this change?
4. If you decided to take a leadership role in initiating change, who would you invite to be part of the change team?

Strong Leadership for Systemic Change

There is good rationale for strong school counselor leadership efforts aimed at addressing at a systemic level concerns like those listed in the Arizona survey. Media accounts suggest similar concerns in schools across the country. A systems perspective takes into account a broader view of a particular problem than a situational perspective and generates systems-level responses. Many reported school counselor concerns address issues for a large number of students and, therefore, are best addressed with a school-wide or community approach. When the school counselor declines to accept the full burden of providing solutions for problems and shares leadership in addressing problems, no one person bears the full weight. In this way, the problems become more manageable. Strong school counselor leadership skills can help counselors share responsibilities in system-wide interventions.

CHAPTER SUMMARY

There is much rationale for school counselor leadership and advocacy. The ASCA standards for school counselors refer to the many leadership activities expected of school counselors. The mandate for school counselor leadership stems from a social justice perspective on education. Current expectations of school counselors in schools and the demands on school counselors are related to current social issues. National data illustrate gaps in academic success among specific groups of students. These gaps in academic success offered examples of targets for system-wide school reform in which school counselors have a leadership role.

Recent research findings support the need to transform the school counseling profession and school counseling education programs to assist school counselors in meeting the needs of students of the 21st century. These findings support school counselors as leaders, advocates, and change agents within schools. National, state, local, and school-specific data offer school counselors and other educational leaders information that assists in the identification of key areas for systemic change. School counselors who stay current with trends in schools and their profession not only maintain an awareness of potential areas for systemic change but also are likely to identify opportunities to lead the way on behalf of their students.

REVIEW AND REFLECT

1. Consider the target problem you identified in the last chapter exercise as you explore responses to the following questions.
    a. What are some of the barriers you and your change team might face as you question the status quo and attempt to initiate change in a school or district?
    b. In a small group, share the target problem you identified and enlist the help of the group to brainstorm some strategies to address and minimize those barriers. Report one or two of your best ideas to the larger group.

RELEVANT WEBSITES

American School Counselor Association: www.schoolcounselor.org
Association for Supervision and Curriculum Development: www.ascd.org
Eye on Education: www.eyeoneducation.com
Reviews of educational policies and practices effective in closing the achievement gap: www.ed.gov/databases/ERIC_Digests/ed460191.html
The Education Trust: www.edtrust.org
The International Center for Leadership in Education: www.daggett.com/
The School Leadership Development Unit: www.sofweb.vic.edu.au/pd/schlead/ http://21stcenturyschools.northcarolina.edu/center

REFERENCES

Baker, S. B., & Gerler, E. R., Jr. (2004). *School counseling for the twenty-first century.* Upper Saddle River, NJ: Pearson Education.

Bolman, L., & Deal, T. (1994). *Becoming a teacher leader: From isolation to collaboration.* Thousand Oaks, CA: Corwin Press.

Braddock, D. (1999). Occupational employment projections to 2008. *Monthly Labor Review, 0098-1818, 122 (11).*

Bradley, L., & Lewis, J. (2000). Introduction. In J. Lewis & L. Bradley (Eds.), *Advocacy in counseling: Counselors, clients and community* (pp. 3–4). Greensboro, NC: ERIC Clearinghouse on Counseling and Student Services.

Education Trust. (1997). *The national guidance and counseling reform program.* Washington, DC: Author.

Education Trust. (1998). *Transforming school counseling initiative* [Brochure].Washington, DC: Author.

Fleetwood, C., & Shelley, K. (2000). The outlook for college graduates, 1998–2008: A balancing act. *Occupational Outlook Quarterly, 0199-4786, 44 (3).*

Garrecht Gassen, S. (September 22, 2004). Charter schools' MAP scores a mixed bag. *Arizona Daily Star.* Tucson, AZ: Star Publishing Co.

Kolodinsky, W., DeVoss, J. A., Brown, L., Montopoli, G., & Moore, M. (2004). Arizona School Counselor Survey, 2004. Paper presented at Arizona School Counselors Association Conference, Mesa, Arizona.

Lee, C. C., & Walz, G. R. (1998). *Social action: A mandate for counselors.* Alexandria, VA: American Counseling Association.

Menacker, J. (1976). Toward a theory of activist guidance. *Personnel and Guidance Journal, 54,* 318–321.

National Center for Educational Statistics. (1999). *National assessment of educational progress, 1999.* Washington, DC: U.S. Department of Education.

Newburger, E. C., & Curry, A. (2000). *Educational attainment in the United States.* Washington, DC: U.S. Department of Commerce, U.S. Census Bureau.

Ponzo, Z. (1974). A counselor and change: Reminiscence and resolutions. *Personnel and Guidance Journal, 53,* 27–32.

Studer, J. R. (2005). *The professional school counselor: An advocate for students.*

U.S. Department of Labor, Bureau of Labor Statistics. (2000). *The outlook for college graduates, 1998–2008.* Washington, DC: Author.

U.S. Department of Labor, Bureau of Labor Statistics. (2000). *Occupational employment projections to 2008.* Washington, DC: Author.

U.S. Department of Census, Bureau of Census Statistics. (March, 2000). Washington, DC: Author.

CHAPTER 4
Leadership Theory for School Counselors

ADDRESSING DIVERSITY ISSUES—A LEADERSHIP CHALLENGE

Eric had been working as a behavioral specialist in a large southwestern school district while he was completing his master's degree in school counseling. During his internship, his professor required that he develop an advocacy project to meet an identified need of the school where he did his internship. He had been asked by the school administration to help a small group of African immigrant children who were having difficulty adjusting to the school environment. Eric began to explore the idea of designing an advocacy project in response to this request.

Eric took some time to observe and interact with the children and their parents. He learned from listening to their stories. He soon realized that typical means of helping children adjust to school would not work in this case. These children came from a radically different background from any of the children in the diverse school and district. In war-torn Sudan, they had lived in refugee camps where they had to scramble for food distributed by humanitarian organizations. Often, the children got only small portions which barely sustained them. In their country, their families were at war with other tribes of their countrymen.

The United Nations Refugee Center helped to resettle these refugees to the United States, where they were able to start a new life. The refugees had a well-founded fear of persecution in their homeland. Sudan has been ravaged by civil war for much of the past 75 years. The war is between the Arab/Muslim majority in

Khartoum and the non-Muslim African rebels in the south. Often, upon arrival in the United States, members of these warring factions would not speak to one another. However, in American schools, all of the Sudanese refugees were categorized as African American under the available demographic descriptors. Except for their racial background, these students had very little in common with the American students of African descent in the schools.

When school district administrators told Eric that 400 additional Sudanese immigrant children would be coming into the school district during the following year, he realized that a proactive systems approach would be necessary to adequately meet the needs of the immigrant children. Eric's advocacy project became more than a learning exercise for his master's degree program. He felt a moral imperative to take action to initiate systemic change on behalf of a population of children in need. He knew that it would take a team effort to effectively assimilate the African immigrant children into his school district and assure their academic, social/personal, and career-planning success. The numerous demands and challenges of the situation prompted him to tap into his own leadership skills and to develop allies and collaborative partnerships with others who had a stake in the success of the immigrant children.

Case Discussion

Questions About This Case

- What were some of the key issues that Eric needed to consider?
- What other options did he have for responding to the challenge of helping the immigrant students?
- How can a school counselor initiate a team effort to address a systemic issue such as the one described in this scenario?
- What messages about school counselor roles and priorities does this scenario convey?
- What can we learn from this case example about working with other personnel in a school?

Further Thoughts on This Case

Eric used an advocacy project assignment in his internship to lay a foundation for a district-wide proactive response to meeting the needs of the African immigrant children in his district. He contacted the director of the center for African American students and discussed his concern about meeting the children's needs. The director encouraged Eric to work with two members of his staff to collect some preliminary data to document the extent of the problem. Eric and his collaborators collected and presented the data to the director of the center for African American students, the district superintendent, and the school board. They also made a number of recommendations based on a review of literature on African immigrant adjustment to life in the United States.

The director of African American students, the superintendent, and the school board were impressed by and appreciative of the team's efforts, the data they collected, and the recommendations made. They passed a motion to retain the collaborative committee, calling it "the African immigrant facilitation team," and charged it with providing in-service training for the administration and faculty of every school in the district to increase awareness of the issues for the African immigrant students and also to make recommendations regarding interventions to assist these students. They also asked the team to collect additional data to monitor the effectiveness of the approaches used to assist the African immigrant students.

CHAPTER OBJECTIVES

The objectives of this chapter are to:

1. Describe a number of contemporary leadership models derived from theories that have influenced the field of educational leadership.
2. Present an integrated leadership model as a viable option for school counselors.

STEPPING UP TO THE PLATE

In the *Handbook of School Counseling*, Cobia and Henderson (2003) address the school counselor's responsibility as an educational leader: "Professional school counselors spend most of each workday developing and maintaining relationships with students, teachers, parents, administrators, and community resource persons. School counselors have unique skills, abilities, and knowledge that enables them to know in which situations to provide leadership and in which situations to support the emergence of leadership in others" (p. 73).

Although it is clear that school counselors function as educational leaders while performing their duties, they typically have not received formal training in educational leadership. They may volunteer out of commitment to their work, or as in Eric's case, administrators within the school or district may "volunteer" them for leadership roles. School counselors may feel poorly prepared for such leadership experiences. While in graduate school, some school counselors may have taken an elective course or two in educational leadership from a department outside of where the school counseling program is housed. Even a limited exposure to leadership theory and/or practices can provide an advantage to the counselor who serves as an active member of a school leadership team. If you are reading this book as part of a course on school counseling leadership, you are probably a member of a new generation of school counselor trainees who is preparing in advance for the call to leadership.

Graduate students and newly graduated counselors typically receive exposure to some hands-on leadership skills during their practicum and internship experiences. Although the experience is valuable, the students are likely to benefit more if they acquire a framework of understanding for the leadership skills and strategies used. School counselor trainees, emerging school-counselor leaders, and all currently practicing school counselors need to further develop leadership skills so that they are ready for the "call to leadership," a mandate that is not negotiable for school counselors of the twenty-first century.

In *Exploring School Counseling*, Tamara Davis (2005) addressed the professional school counselor as leader: "Developing leadership skills in school counselors is of the utmost importance. Without the ability to use leadership skills at the most opportune time and in an appropriate manner, many opportunities for positive change can be lost. The students, their families, and the community are the recipients of the benefits of school counselors with strong leadership skills" (p. 220).

Defining and Describing Leadership

Finish the sentences, "Leadership is _____" and "Leadership is not _____" with as many descriptors as you can list. Keep this list available as you review the rest of the chapter. Compare your list with the descriptors addressed by the authors.

Leadership is

_____

_____

_____

Leadership is not

_____

_____

_____

LEADERSHIP EXPECTATIONS OF SCHOOL COUNSELORS

After an extensive review of current literature (Adelman & Taylor, 2002; Bemak, 2000; Bemak & Cornely, 2002; Dahir, 2001; Gysbers & Henderson, 2000, 2001; Hatch & Bowers, 2002; House & Hayes, 2002; Keys, 2000; and Rowley, Sink, & MacDonald, 2002), Baker and Gerler (2004) summarized twenty-nine leadership behaviors expected of school counselors. Box 4-1 presents a condensed version of the list to highlight key school counselor leadership behaviors in ten categories.

The expected leadership behaviors of school counselors presented in Box 4-1 imply that school counselors understand and know how to apply a variety of leadership skills to myriad problems. For example, school counselors are expected to have knowledge and skills for effective program development and maintenance. They need to maintain awareness of current needs, issues, resources, and opportunities. They must be skilled in public relations, group facilitation, collaboration and consultation, and conflict resolution. They are expected to be versed in data collection and reporting and to be effective in their communications with various members of the school and local community. School counselors can better address these expectations in a meaningful and systematic manner if they possess an understanding of leadership models and applications.

Box 4-1   Expected School Counselor Leadership Behaviors

1. Developing and maintaining a comprehensive school counseling program aligned with the mission of the school
2. Forming and leading relevant school committees, conducting meetings, developing and committing to action plans
3. Promoting the counseling program, educating and involving others in the mission of the school and the counseling program
4. Developing support systems within the school and district; supporting, collaborating, and consulting with other school personnel, for example, teachers, school psychologists, nurses, and social workers
5. Mediating conflicts, effectively utilizing group process knowledge and skills, and employing multicultural sensitivity in problem solving
6. Identifying and utilizing opportunities for empowerment and building a sense of community by partnering, building consensus, and collaborating with diverse groups of stakeholders
7. Developing and maintaining an awareness of current needs of students, bringing in and coordinating community services for students, and developing mutual prevention/intervention programs with community agencies
8. Developing and maintaining a crisis response team
9. Collecting and sharing data regarding the comprehensive school counseling program
10. Informing administrators about the comprehensive school counseling plan, including goals and objectives, and providing timely updates on its progress

Adapted from Baker and Gerler, 2004.

Self-Assessment and Exploration

In this exercise you will assess your preparedness for performing leadership behaviors.

A. Rating Your Preparedness

Instructions: Review the ten leadership behavior categories in Box 4-1 and score yourself for each item on a scale of 1–10 based on your competence level, where 1 = completely unprepared and 10 = completely prepared. A score between 1 and 5 indicates a sense of being unprepared; the lower the score, the lower your sense of competence. A score between 6 and 8 indicates a sense of competence in that leadership behavior. A score of 8 to 10 indicates a high level of perceived competence in that leadership behavior category. The maximum total score for all items is 100.

Expected Leadership Behavior	Your Competence Score (Circle one number for each behavior) Unprepared ⟵ ⟶ Prepared
1. Development of a comprehensive school counseling program	1 2 3 4 5 6 7 8 9 10
2. Formation/facilitation of school committees and meetings	1 2 3 4 5 6 7 8 9 10
3. Education of others on the counseling program mission	1 2 3 4 5 6 7 8 9 10
4. Development of school and district support systems	1 2 3 4 5 6 7 8 9 10
5. Culturally sensitive conflict mediation and problem solving	1 2 3 4 5 6 7 8 9 10
6. Maximization of empowerment and community-building opportunities	1 2 3 4 5 6 7 8 9 10
7. Coordination of community services and partnered development of prevention/intervention programs	1 2 3 4 5 6 7 8 9 10
8. Development of a crisis response team and plan	1 2 3 4 5 6 7 8 9 10
9. Collection and reporting of school counseling program data	1 2 3 4 5 6 7 8 9 10
10. Communication with administrators regarding the school counseling plan	1 2 3 4 5 6 7 8 9 10
Total Competence Score	_____

B. Identifying Your Strengths and Areas for Improvement

You can use the following scale to determine your overall perceived competence in school counseling leadership behaviors. You will also want to consider your scores on individual items to determine areas in which you have strengths and areas for improvement.

Instructions: Circle the items with scores lower than 6 for use in a later chapter exercise when you develop a leadership improvement plan.

Competent	80–100
Somewhat competent	60–80
Unprepared for leadership	1–59

LEADERSHIP THEORIES AND MODELS

Educational leadership models have been greatly influenced by the fields of psychology and social psychology. This section explores six current leadership models: Situational Leadership, Transformational Leadership, Moral Leadership, the Learning Organization, Servant Leadership, and Empowered Leadership.

Because of the overlap of psychological theories with most educational leadership theories, concepts from a number of leadership theories can be integrated compatibly into an educational leadership model that is a better fit for school counselors than any one of these models. Later in this chapter, we incorporate leadership concepts described here into such an integrated model.

Situational Leadership Model (Based on Situational Theory)

Hersey and Blanchard crafted the Situational Leadership Model in the late 1960s (Hersey & Blanchard, 1969; Hersey, 1984). Through their research they developed a leadership model that focuses on adapting leadership approaches to situational demands, requiring that the leader assess the readiness level of those being asked to complete a task. The two major components of readiness are ability and willingness (Hersey, 1984). Ability has to do with one's knowledge, experience, and skill. Willingness has to do with one's confidence, commitment, and motivation.

This model also describes two dimensions of leadership behavior: Task Behavior and Relationship Behavior. The style used by the leader depends on the readiness level of the group or individuals assigned to the task. In the Task Behavior style, the leader explains what is to be done, how it is to be done, and when the task is to be completed. In the Relationship Behavior style, the leader is supportive and acts in a more facilitative manner than a directive manner in the completion of the task.

Transformational Leadership Models (Based on Transformational Leadership Theory)

Transformational Leadership Theory views the leader as a change agent who shares his/her vision and inspires others. According to this model, a good leader focuses on building relationships and believes in participative leadership. Two of the best-known transformational leadership approaches are W. Edwards Deming's model (1993) and Warren Bennis's model (1994).

Deming's Total Quality Management Leadership Model

Deming's Total Quality Management leadership model (Deming, 1993) emphasizes 14 points (see Box 4-2). Deming emphasizes focusing on process, including the activities of teaching and learning, classroom climate, curriculum, and relationships within the school environment. He believed that quality in these relationships leads to high-quality outcomes. Deming developed his model primarily to revamp management approaches in industry, but it has been applied to education as well.

Sergiovanni (2001) criticized Deming's philosophy as an example of one that can cause confusion. Deming espouses "Total Quality Management." However, the word *quality* is rarely used in Deming's writing and the concept of totally managing is not part of his philosophy. Instead, he promotes not managing for control but rather the idea of honoring variation. Deming believes that his fourteen principles must be applied as a whole, including not using slogans like "TQM" (Total Quality Management). Yet, if his fourteen points were followed completely, many well-established procedures in schools, like testing, grading, evaluation, and rankings would be dropped. No Child Left Behind legislation makes the adoption of

---

Box 4-2   Deming's (1993) Fourteen Points of Total Quality Management

1. Create constancy of purpose for the improvement of product and service.
2. Adopt the new philosophy.
3. Cease dependence on mass inspection.
4. End the practice of awarding business on price tag alone.
5. Constantly improve the system of production and service.
6. Institute training.
7. Institute leadership.
8. Drive out fear.
9. Break down barriers between staff areas.
10. Eliminate slogans, exhortations, and targets for the workforce.
11. Eliminate numerical quotas.
12. Remove barriers to pride of workmanship.
13. Institute a vigorous education and retraining program.
14. Take action to accomplish the transformation.

Adapted from Deming, 1993.

---

this transformational model as a whole by American schools unfeasible. Yet many of Deming's ideas have been applied by educational leaders who share a similar philosophy while feeling pressured to conform to contradictory institutionalized policies and procedures.

Bennis's Transformational Leadership Model

In the Transformational Leadership Model of Bennis (1994), leadership is conceptualized as full expression of oneself. Bennis stated: "Well, what's become clear to me . . . is that for leaders and organizations to succeed, there are three basic ingredients for success. And if I were restricted to three words in any commencement speech, they would be ideas, relationships, and adventure" (Bennis, 1994, p. xiv). Bennis explained that *ideas* are for change. *Relationships* refer to harmonious and open interactions, empowerment, and a sense of inclusion among all who work together. *Adventure* refers to active risk, curiosity, and challenge.

Effective leaders are able to express themselves, to know their strengths and weaknesses, and to manage them effectively, according to Bennis. Good leaders know what they want and how to communicate it, how to achieve goals, and how to get the cooperation and support of others. Leaders are people in whom "life is the career" (Bennis, 1994, p. 4). The twenty-eight leaders Bennis interviewed for his book *On Becoming a Leader* (1994) agreed that leaders are made, that they continue growing and learning to express themselves throughout their lives. Effective leaders are adult learners in charge of their learning and their way of living.

According to Bennis (1994), becoming a leader is a transformational process. Good leaders think about what is best for their organization for the long term while making it look good in the short term. Bennis believed that there are unlimited opportunities and challenges for leaders. Good leaders have vision and character that guide the leader in doing the right thing. Leaders master the context. They do this by becoming self-expressive, listening to their inner voice, learning from the right mentors, and giving themselves over to a guiding vision. "Where there is no vision, the people perish" (Proverbs 29:18).

Bennis (1994) identified four basic leadership ingredients: a guiding vision of what the leader wants to do professionally and personally; passion for life, vocation, and course of action; integrity that includes self-knowledge, candor, and maturity, and is the basis of trust; and curiosity and daring (p. 39). He stated that leadership courses teach only skills. The leader must learn character and vision outside of the classroom. Leadership includes "innovative learning" (p. 76) with the components of active and imaginative anticipation, listening to others, participation in shaping events, and self-direction.

Bennis (1994) made a distinction between leaders and managers. Managers administer whereas leaders innovate. Managers imitate whereas leaders originate. Managers accept the status quo whereas leaders challenge it. Managers ask, "how and when?" Leaders ask, "what and why?" Managers have their eyes on the bottom line whereas leaders watch the horizon. Managers do things right. The leader does the right thing. Bennis contended that effective leaders move away from "square hats" to "sombreros," away from traditional linear thinking to the use of synthesis and imagination. Becoming a leader is becoming oneself and separating who one is from what the world thinks one is. Similar distinctions have been made between the traditional and the new-vision description of school counselors (Education Trust, 2003).

Bennis's (1994) four lessons of self-knowledge include: recognizing that a person is his/her own best teacher; accepting responsibility; realizing that one can learn whatever one wants to learn; and reflecting on experience as the way to true understanding. It is important to reflect on the impact of childhood and significant others on one's development. Leaders reflect on how and whether they have resolved Eric Erikson's eight developmental crises. They recognize that healthy resolutions to these conflicts lead to healthy psychological functioning that includes hope, autonomy, purpose, competence, integrity, empathy, maturity, and wisdom.

Psychologist Alfred Adler emphasized internal influences on behavior, including a person's values, beliefs, and attitudes. Similarly, Bennis noted that leaders can use the internal influence of their thinking to change their understanding of the past and its effect on their behavior. He quoted Socrates: "The unexamined life is not worth living" (1994, p. 68). Bennis added his own insight, "The unexamined life is impossible to live successfully" (1994, p. 68). Leaders need to make their lives their own. They can only do that by themselves. In their graduate training, school counselors become skilled in helping students to utilize internal experiences to influence behavior: Students' thoughts are used to influence behavior.

Effective leaders take a whole-brain approach to leading, in which they listen to their "inner voice" (Bennis, 1994, p. 105). Leaders learn to lead by leading. They generate trust by being constant, congruent, reliable, and demonstrating integrity. They are flexible, creative, and proactive and learn from experience. They not only accept change and ambiguity but even thrive on it. Effective leaders create learning organizations that effectively cope with change. They promote and manage the dream, embrace error, and encourage reflective backtalk and dissent. They possess optimism, faith, and hope. Educational leaders understand the Pygmalian effect, in which they get what they expect from others.

Effective leaders have a sense of the future and develop the patience to make long-term plans. They are conscious of "stakeholder symmetry" (p. 200), work to balance competing claims of various stakeholders, and create strategic alliances. Effective leaders demonstrate competence, strategic thinking, and the ability to synthesize all means of expression. Leaders need to learn how to *be* in order to know how to *do*. Everything the leader does reflects the leader's self. Becoming a transformational leader can be viewed as a lifelong developmental process of becoming fully oneself. This process can be compared to the concept of self-actualization associated with Maslow (1968) and Carl Rogers (1980) that refers to the basic human drive toward growth, completeness, and fulfillment.

Moral Leadership

Thomas J. Sergiovanni (1992) is a leading researcher and author on moral leadership. His work indicates that the leader who believes in the Moral Leadership Theory is motivating, spends time explaining and teaching, and works at achieving workable unity. Sergiovanni (1992) describes a model of leadership that connects the interactions between the heart, the head, and the hand. The model starts with the heart (what one values and believes), that interacts with the head (one's mental picture of how the world works) that leads to the hand (one's decisions, actions, and behaviors).

Sergiovanni (1992) emphasized the importance of the sacred dimension of leadership. His theory is considered a moral leadership theory. He emphasized building a sense of community in schools. By incorporating the concept of "servant leadership" into his model, his theory and model also fall into the category of servant leadership. The concepts of a sense of community and servant leadership are similar to the Adlerian counseling theory concepts of social interest and the need to belong. Greenleaf (1977) is credited with the servant leadership concept and defines it as the way in which leaders gain legitimacy for their roles as leaders.

Leadership, according to Sergiovanni (1992, 2001), is both a form of behavior and a form of stewardship. In morally responsive school communities, teachers, counselors, and principals are stewards and servants with shared values, commitment, and a sense of empowerment concerning duties and obligations. Leadership is shared by everyone in the community of learners. The community members focus on a common vision rather than seeking to follow one person as leader. Community members become self-managers and followers in alignment with the common values and vision of the learning community.

Sergiovanni (1992) stated that educators could be more successful in school improvement by providing substitutes for direct leadership. Examples of leadership substitutes include responsiveness to a learning community's norms and the associated work, collegiality, intrinsically motivating work, and commitment to the professional ideal of educational professionals.

Sergiovanni (1992, 2001) suggested reinventing and expanding the concept of leadership to include a moral dimension, which includes factors such as emotions, group membership, meaning, morality, intuition, and obligation. He believed that leadership should be based on professional and moral authority. This type of leadership is balanced by connecting process with substance. The effective leader experiences a connection and interaction of his/her values (heart), his/her mental pictures of the world (head), and his/her decision and actions (hand). Like Bennis, Sergiovanni contends that moral leaders focus on "doing the right things" instead of "doing things right" (p. 4).

Like other leadership-model architects, Sergiovanni believes that leadership comes from within. He points out the limitations of the old adage "What gets rewarded gets done," and suggests replacing it with "What is rewarding gets done," or "What we believe in gets done" (p. 26). In the latter situations, work gets done without careful monitoring because the work provides opportunities for challenge, meaning, discovery, variety, feelings of achievement, and responsibility. The work provides for an experience of "flow" (Csikzentmihalyi, 1997), a state in which work is intrinsically motivating.

In describing the experience of "flow," Csikzentmihalyi (1997) explained the meaning of an associated word, *autotelic*, as it refers to activities and to personality. Autotelic is a word composed of two Greek roots: *auto* (self), and *telos* (goal). An autotelic activity is one that is done for its own sake because to experience it is the main goal. For instance, if I played a game of chess primarily to enjoy the game, that game would be an autotelic experience for me; whereas if I played for money or to achieve a competitive ranking in the chess world, the same game would be primarily *exotelic*, that is, motivated by an outside goal. Applied to personality, autotelic denotes an individual who generally does things for their own sake rather than to achieve some later external goal (p. 117).

An autotelic person needs very little in terms of material goods and creature comforts because the activities of the person's life are already sufficiently rewarding and a source of the experience of flow for that person. The autotelic person is a wellspring of psychic energy that is focused on learning, empathizing, and continuously growing through acceptance of challenges and risks. This type of person is less focused on him- or herself and more involved in enjoying and caring about even the routine aspects of life. This description of flow and the autotelic person clarifies Sergiovanni's concept of leadership from within.

People generally experience flow in exceptional moments in life when they have a sense of effortlessness in their actions. The experience usually occurs when the goals are clear and the rules for action are understood. There is no need to question what one needs to do. Flow occurs when both the challenges faced and the person's skills are high. "When goals are clear, feedback relevant, and challenges and skills are in balance, attention becomes ordered and fully invested" (Csikzentmihalyi, 1990, p. 31).

Sergiovanni (1992) described five characteristics of the virtuous school. The virtuous school, as an organization, believes that it must become a learning community with teachers, counselors, and administrators who are servant leaders. The virtuous school subscribes to the belief that every student can learn, and the learning community works toward that end. The virtuous school seeks to serve the whole student and honors respect. The parents, teachers, community, and school are partners. These characteristics serve as a foundation for policy structure for the school.

The Learning Organization Model

The Fifth Discipline (Senge, 1990), also known as the Learning Organization Model, focuses on five disciplines that overcome "organizational learning disabilities." This approach to leadership maintains a continuous feedback process to foster learning for improvement of the entire organization. Senge utilizes science, psychology, management theory, and spiritual wisdom for his model.

He describes five disciplines. The first discipline is *personal mastery*, which includes personal growth and learning through competence, skills, spiritual growth, creativity in viewing life, and a personal vision of one's life purpose. The second discipline is *mental models,* which involves managing one's internal images of how the world works. The third discipline is a *shared vision,* which is "a force in people's hearts" connecting them in learning and work. The fourth discipline is *team learning,* in which a group functions as a whole, with a shared vision and synergy of efforts. The fifth discipline is *systems thinking,* which integrates the other disciplines and keeps a view of the big picture and of the interrelationships of all of the disciplines. In a learning organization, people recognize that they are connected to the organization and that they affect the world. Senge's model is comprehensive and contains many useful and teachable concepts for school counselors.

Servant Leadership

Stephen Covey (1991) and Sergiovanni (1992) were two contributors to the Servant Leadership Model. This section focuses on Covey's description of the behaviors to be practiced by those who aspire to be servant leaders. According to Covey, the servant leader serves first and leads second. The servant leader believes in the human spirit and leads by moral principles. This theory also focuses on participating in actions that build trust and nurture the growth and development of the individual.

Covey's book *Principle-Centered Leadership* (1991) offers a framework focused on relationships, both personal and professional. The servant leadership model described in Covey's book represents the achievement of balance among family, personal, and professional life. Such balance is exactly what school counselors hope to facilitate in their own lives and in the lives of their students and their students' families.

Covey's (1991) leadership model is based on eight characteristics of principle-centered leaders. This type of leadership is developed from within and is practiced on four levels: personal, in relation to oneself; interpersonal, in relationships with others; managerial, in accepting responsibility to get a job done with others; and organizational, in needing to organize people. Eight characteristics define the principle-centered leader.

Servant leaders can be characterized as continually learning. They care about the needs of others and are service-oriented. They have a positive outlook and radiate positive energy. Servant leaders believe in other people. They see life as an adventure and are willing to take some risks. They are synergistic, believing the whole is more than the sum of its parts. In addition, they take care of themselves by exercising for self-renewal. They lead balanced lives. School leaders who live by these principles create environments in which others thrive and are empowered to develop their leadership potential.

Covey recommended, in his book *The 7 Habits of Highly Effective People* (1989), that individuals "begin with the end in mind." He described ways to develop a personal or organizational mission statement. This type of statement helps leaders understand their destination. It helps leaders know where they are going, and it keeps them from getting involved in a flurry of directionless activity, working hard but not efficiently or effectively. Effective school counseling programs have well-conceived mission statements, which clarify the steps needed to achieve goals.

With a clear mission statement, leaders can develop a vivid mental picture of the better future they envision. Covey (1989) emphasized the principle "all things are created twice," which means that before leaders realize their goals, there is a mental picture that precedes the physical creation. In order to build a building, one should imagine it first in great detail before ever picking up a shovel and digging on the actual building site.

School counselors can apply the concepts of "beginning with the end in mind," a mission statement, and "all things are created twice" to their personal lives as well as to their professional lives in working with children. They can develop their own mission statement to guide their steps toward their vision of a better future. Some school counselors have separate professional and personal mission statements. Others have one broad mission statement that covers all aspects of their lives.

To guide the development of a professional mission statement, counselors can align their own statement with the mission of the state department of education, their school district's guidance mission statement, and their school's general mission and guidance-specific mission.

A good way to develop a personal mission statement is through a reflective process. Covey recommends beginning by examining one's roles in life and the contributions for which one would like to be remembered in each key role. He suggests considering what characteristics, values, and principles are represented in those contributions. This provides a good source of material for a mission statement. The statement should be inspiring and empowering. It should represent the best of a person's inner life and the fulfillment of gifts in all realms of life. It should have as its basis a sense of contribution and higher purpose and should align with the person's vision and values. An example of a mission statement is: My mission is to fully develop my potential and to facilitate the same in others.

Developing a Personal Mission Statement

Develop a personal mission statement organized around the following steps. (Use the space provided or a separate sheet of paper.)

1. In the first column, list all of the roles you fill in your life.
2. In the second column, list the contributions for which you would like to be remembered for each role.
3. In the third column, list the related values, characteristics, and principles represented in the contributions column.

The roles you fill in your life	Contributions for which you would like to be remembered	Values, characteristics, and principles represented in your contributions
_____	_____	_____
_____	_____	_____
_____	_____	_____
_____	_____	_____
_____	_____	_____
_____	_____	_____
_____	_____	_____
_____	_____	_____
_____	_____	_____
_____	_____	_____
_____	_____	_____
_____	_____	_____
_____	_____	_____
_____	_____	_____
_____	_____	_____
_____	_____	_____

4. Review what you have written and summarize your mission in a statement that is inspiring and empowering and that represents a sense of contribution and higher purpose that aligns with your vision and values. Post your mission statement in your meeting room for the entire group to see. It represents public acknowledgement of your mission. Put a copy of your mission statement in a prominent place and review it often.

Empowerment Leadership Theory

Studies on the Empowerment Leadership Theory conducted by Kouzes and Posner (1995) and Warren Bennis (1994) found that the most effective leaders accept input from others, designate power to others, and motivate individuals to achieve individual success. Bennis's leadership model was described in detail in the section on Transformational Leadership. His approach contains concepts that fit in both the Transformational Leadership and Empowerment Leadership categories.

The Leadership Challenge model of Kouzes and Posner (1995) emphasizes the human need to be respected and acknowledged as a source of motivation. This empowerment leadership model includes five practices and ten commitments of effective leaders. The model is based on more than ten years of personal-best cases of leaders who were able to lead others to accomplish extraordinary things. The five practices and their corresponding commitments are listed here.

Challenging the process is the first practice, and the related commitments are to search out challenges and take risks. The second practice is *inspiring a shared vision,* and the commitments are envisioning an uplifting future and enlisting others in a common vision. The third practice is *enabling others to act.* The two commitments corresponding to this practice are to foster collaboration and strengthen people by giving away power and providing support. The fourth practice of the Kouzes and Posner approach is to *model the way.* The related commitments are to set the example by acting in ways that are consistent with shared values and promoting small victories for continued progress. The fifth practice is *encouraging the heart.* The related commitments are to recognize individual contributions and celebrate team accomplishments.

The Leadership Challenge model was designed to develop leadership in everyone. It addresses self-development, self-improvement, and empowerment. Kouzes and Posner (1995) developed a leadership assessment instrument called the Leadership Practices Inventory (LPI), described in Chapter 6. The Leadership Challenge self-improvement journey begins with the LPI assessment, review, and analysis of the results, development of action plans, and ongoing behavioral changes as the leader continuously develops as an effective leader.

Self-Assessment and Exploration

This is a group exercise we call the Jigsaw Puzzle.

Materials Needed: At least one copy of *The Leadership Challenge* (Kouzes & Posner, 1995) for each group of five participants.

Instructions: Divide into groups of five. (If there are four members in one group, one person can serve in place of two or one person from another group of five can divide time between the two groups.)

1. Assign each member of the group to read a different section of *The Leadership Challenge,* according to the five practices. Each member of the group is responsible for reading the section on his/her assigned practice and associated commitments.
2. Group members are responsible for learning about their assigned leadership practice and commitments and preparing to explain them to their group, relating them to school counseling practice.
3. Participants meet in their groups with any notes needed to briefly explain the practice and commitments assigned to them. When all group members understand one practice, the next group member presents his/her assigned practice and commitments. The process continues until each group member presents and the group understands all five practices and commitments.
4. When all groups have completed the small-group exercise, meet in the larger group and discuss how well the Leadership Challenge practices can serve new-vision school counselors, their students, students' parents, and colleagues.

AN INTEGRATED SCHOOL COUNSELING LEADERSHIP MODEL

A balanced framework can be developed by integrating key concepts from counseling theories and leadership models reviewed in the previous sections. A systematic integration of relevant aspects of theories from each area can offer a practical, understandable leadership model for school counselors. When the theoretical concepts and framework are clarified, the applications follow smoothly.

There are numerous overlapping and complementary concepts in counseling and leadership theory. For example, most counseling theories emphasize relationships. Such an emphasis fits well with leadership concepts that include the following:

- servant leadership
- systems thinking
- the learning organization
- moral leadership
- person-centered leadership
- principle-centered leadership
- empowerment concepts

Rogers's (1959, 1980) concept of self-actualization can be compared with Bennis's (1994) description of an effective leader's full self-expression. Bennis also emphasizes harmonious and open interactions, empowerment, and a sense of inclusion, which are concepts frequently used by counselors of various theoretical orientations.

The Integrated School Counseling Leadership Model, as presented in the next section, demonstrates how well key concepts from the various leadership theories and models combine to form a meaningful and practical framework for school counselors as educational leaders. This integrated model translates smoothly from theory to application for school counselor educational leaders in K–12 educational settings. The philosophy, behavior, and leadership characteristics of the model emphasize an approach to school counselor leadership that facilitates the work outlined for school counselors in the American School Counselor National Model.

Box 4-3 highlights key concepts from the leadership theories and models reviewed in this chapter. The concepts are generally compatible and fairly easily incorporated into a more comprehensive integrated school counselor leadership model that applies to the effective performance of the duties of a professional school counselor. Listed in Box 4-4 are principles of effective school counselor leadership based on an integrative leadership model that borrows from the numerous leadership models reviewed in this chapter.

The Integrative Model for School Counseling Leadership concepts presented in Box 4-3 and behaviors in Box 4-4 incorporate a continuous self-improvement process (Bennis, 1994) through lifelong learning (Covey, 1991). It is a process of becoming oneself and fully expressing oneself (Bennis, 1994) and self-actualizing (Rogers, 1959, 1980; Maslow, 1968). Effective school counseling leaders engage in ongoing self-reflection (Bennis, 1994) as they develop as leaders from the inside out.

Self-Assessment and Exploration

In this exercise you will compare expected school counselor leadership behaviors with integrated leadership model behaviors.

Box 4-3   Leadership Concepts Incorporated into the Integrated School
Counseling Leadership Model

Leadership Philosophy	Servant leadership—leaders serve first and lead second
	Leadership from within—start with knowledge of core values from within
	Moral leadership—develop a new philosophy that connects heart, head, and hand
	Learning organizations—team learning starts with a shared vision
	Transformational process—leaders view life of continuous learning for self-expression
	Situational leadership—adapt leadership approaches to situational demands
Leadership Behaviors	Doing the right thing
	Forming strategic alliances
	Forming supportive, harmonious, open relationships
	Breaking down barriers, driving out fear
	Being adventurous, an active risk-taker, facing challenges
	Practicing effective communication
	Collaborating and cooperating
	Innovating
	Originating
	Challenging the status quo
	Asking what and why
	Taking a whole-brain approach
	Balancing short-term versus long-term objectives
	Having a guiding vision, with a clear sense of future
	Being goal-oriented, with constancy of purpose
	Listening to the inner voice
	Practicing continual growth
	Learning by experience
	Finding the right mentors
Leadership Characteristics	Passion for life (autotelic personality)
	Integrity
	Curiosity and daring
	Concern for doing the right thing
	Desire to be a lifelong learner
	Self-directed
	Idea generator for change
	Thrives on change
	Systems thinker

DeVoss, 2004.

Instructions: In small groups, identify the integrated leadership model behaviors in Box 4-4 relevant to each of the ten expected leadership behaviors of school counselors described in Box 4-1 and listed below. Next to each behavior, circle one or more of the letters most relevant to the items in Box 4-4. Make notes to which you can refer in the exercise in Chapter 7 in which you will develop a leadership improvement plan.

Box 4-4   Integrative School Counselor Leadership Model Behaviors

---

a. Develop leadership from within based on values and life principles.

b. Live with integrity and demonstrate character and morality by doing the right things instead of striving to do things right. Leaders listen to their inner voice and reject superficial efforts at school transformation that lack moral imperative.

c. Learn by experience and reflection and continue to grow as self-directed adult learners who use a whole-brain approach to process information.

d. Value and promote harmonious relationships through cultural competence, celebration of differences, social interest, and service to others.

e. Advocate for social justice.

f. Model a democratic way of supporting the American School Counselor Association's guiding vision through shared leadership opportunities that encourage contributions to the learning community and foster experience of belonging, power, freedom, and fun.

g. Believe in collaboration and are skilled in developing supportive and cooperative strategic alliances.

h. Seek mentors who have positive values and philosophy.

i. Facilitate conditions of trust, open and effective communication, and opportunities for positive growth and self-actualization.

j. Follow first and believe in a guiding vision associated with mental pictures.

k. Share commitment with other educational leaders to the school's guiding vision for transformation of the school.

l. View life as an adventure, life as career; take active risks, seek challenges.

m. Demonstrate passion for life with curiosity and daring.

n. Thrive on change and challenging the status quo, asking what and why.

o. Utilize systems thinking and develop interdependent relationships that promote the school's guiding vision.

p. Use contracts that support accountability and responsibility in achieving measurable goals and collect objective data.

Expected Leadership Behaviors from Box 4-1	*Integrated Model Behaviors from Box 4-4*
1. Development of a comprehensive school counseling program	a b c d e f g h i j k l m n o p
2. Formation/facilitation of school committees and meetings	a b c d e f g h i j k l m n o p

Expected Leadership Behaviors from Box 4-1	Integrated Model Behaviors from Box 4-4
3. Education of others on the counseling program mission	a b c d e f g h i j k l m n o p
4. Development of school and district support systems	a b c d e f g h i j k l m n o p
5. Culturally sensitive conflict mediation and problem solving	a b c d e f g h i j k l m n o p
6. Maximization of empowerment and community-building opportunities	a b c d e f g h i j k l m n o p
7. Coordination of community services and partnered development of prevention/intervention programs	a b c d e f g h i j k l m n o p
8. Development of a crisis response team and plan	a b c d e f g h i j k l m n o p
9. Collection and sharing of school counseling program data	a b c d e f g h i j k l m n o p

Expected Leadership Behaviors from Box 4-1	*Integrated Model Behaviors from Box 4-4*
10. Communication with administrators about the school counseling plan	a b c d e f g h i j k l m n o p

Following this review and integration of educational leadership theories, it is useful to pause, reflect for a moment, and gain some perspective with assistance from Heider's *The Tao of Leadership* (1986), a book of quotes from Lao Tzu. The following was taken from a section titled "Unclutter Your Mind."

Beginners acquire new theories and techniques until their minds are cluttered with options. Advanced students forget their many options. They allow the theories and techniques that they have learned to recede into the background. Learn to unclutter your mind. Learn to simplify your work. As you rely less and less on knowing just what to do, your work will become more direct and more powerful (p. 95).

CHAPTER SUMMARY

A number of contemporary leadership models have influenced the field of educational leadership. Some of the currently popular models include the Situational Model of Hersey and Blanchard, the Transformational Model of Bennis and Deming, the Moral Model of Sergiovanni, the Learning Organization Model of Senge, the Servant Leadership Model of Covey, and the Empowerment Models of Bennis and of Kouzes and Posner. An integrated model of leadership that incorporates many dimensions of leadership required of effective school counselors, such as the one proposed in this chapter, is likely to be more comprehensive and a better fit for school counselors than any one leadership model alone. School counselors need a wide array of leadership behaviors available to them as they address the many challenges facing them on a day-to-day basis. Understanding theories and models of leadership is useful in articulating one's leadership approach. However, as Bennis (1994) emphasized, leaders learn to lead by leading. School counselors need practice in applying leadership skills and developing their own unique leadership styles.

REVIEW AND REFLECT

1. Using your book, a self-reflection journal or on a separate sheet of paper address the following questions that were adapted from Bennis (1994, p. 7).
   a. What do you believe are notable leadership qualities that you possess?

_____

_____

_____

b. What experiences have been vital to your leadership development to this point?

_____

_____

_____

_____

_____

c. What impact do you believe failure has on leadership development?

_____

_____

_____

_____

_____

d. What are your earliest recollections of leadership behavior?

_____

_____

_____

_____

_____

e. Who are the leaders in your life, or in general, whom you particularly admire?

_____

_____

_____

_____

_____

f. What can organizations do to encourage or stifle leaders?

_____

_____

_____

_____

_____

2. As a group, with one person guiding, do some deep breathing and muscle relaxation (adapt as appropriate for participants with limitations for this activity). Sit in a relaxed position with arms and legs uncrossed. Inhale and hold your breath for a few seconds. Then slowly release and say the word *relax* as you exhale. Do this breathing exercise once or twice more. Follow this by tensing and relaxing at least a few muscle groups, for example, making fists, then relaxing your fingers and pulling your shoulders up to your ears and then letting them down slowly. Continue breathing in a relaxed manner.

   Then close your eyes and think back to a time in your life when you experienced "flow" (Csikzentmihalyi, 1997), a state in which your work or play was intrinsically motivating. When your "journey" ends, take a few moments to draw a picture that represents that experience. It can be a literal drawing, such as a drawing of yourself picking apples, or a metaphorical representation, such as a rainbow or a unique combination of shapes and/or colors. Write about key aspects of that experience that contributed to flow. With a learning partner, share what you would like to about your memory of flow.

_____

_____

_____

_____

_____

_____

_____

_____

_____

_____

_____

_____

_____

_____

_____

_____

_____

RELEVANT WEBSITES

American Association of School Administrators: www.aasa.org/

American School Counselor Association: www.schoolcounselor.org

Association for Supervision and Curriculum Development: www.ascd.org

Eye on Education: www.eyeoneducation.com

National Association of Secondary School Principals:
www.principals.org/www.questia.com/

Reviews of educational policies and practices effective in closing the achievement
gap: www.ed.gov/databases/ERIC_Digests/ed460191.html

The Education Trust: www.edtrust.org

The International Center for Leadership in Education: www.daggett.com/

The School Leadership Development Unit: www.sofweb.vic.edu.au/pd/schlead/
http://21stcenturyschools.northcarolina.edu/center

REFERENCES

Adelman, H. S., & Taylor, L. (2002). School counselors and school reform: New directions. *Professional School Counseling, 5*, 235–248.

Baker, S. B., & Gerler, E. R., Jr. (2004). *School counseling for the twenty-first century.* Upper Saddle River, NJ: Pearson Education.

Bemak, F. (2000). Transforming the role of the counselor to provide leadership in educational reform through collaboration. *Professional School Counseling, 3*, 323–331.

Bemak, F., & Cornely, L. (2002). The SAFI model as a critical link between marginalized families and schools: A literature review and strategies for school counselors. *Journal of Counseling & Development, 5*, 322–331.

Bennis, W. (1994). *On becoming a leader.* Cambridge, MA: Perseus Books.

Bensimon, E. M., Neuman, A., & Birnbaum, R. (1989). Making sense of administrative leadership: The "L" word in higher education (ASHE-ERIC Higher Education No. 1). Washington, DC: George Washington University, School of Education and Human Development.

Bracey, G. W. (2004). The 14th Bracey report on the condition of public education. *Phi Delta Kappan, 86*(2), 149–167.

Cobia, D. C., & Henderson, D. A. (2003). *Handbook of school counseling.* Upper Saddle River, NJ: Merrill Prentice Hall.

Covey, S. R. (1989). *The 7 habits of highly effective people.* New York: Simon and Schuster.

Covey, S. R. (1991). *Principle-centered leadership.* New York: Summit Books.

Csikzentmihalyi, M. (1997). *Finding flow.* New York: Basic Books.

Dahir, C. (2001). The national standards for school counseling programs: Development and implementation. *Professional School Counseling, 4*, 320–327.

Davis, T. (2005). *Exploring school counseling: Professional practices and perspectives.* Boston: Lahaska Press.

Deming, W. E. (1993). *The new economics for industry, government, and education.* Cambridge, MA: MIT Press.

Education Trust. (2003). *Transforming school counseling initiative* [Brochure]. Washington, DC: Author.

Greenleaf, R. K. (1977). *Servant leadership: A journey into the nature of legitimate power and greatness.* New York: Paulist.

Gysbers, N. C., & Henderson, P. (2000). *Developing and managing your school guidance program* (3rd ed.). Alexandria, VA: American Counseling Association.

Gysbers, N. C., & Henderson, P. (2001). Comprehensive guidance and counseling programs: A rich history and a bright future. *Professional School Counseling, 4*, 246–256.

Hatch, T., & Bowers, J. (2002, May/June). The block to build on. *ASCA Counselor,* 13–17.

Heider, J. (1986). *The tao of leadership.* New York: Bantam Books.

Hersey, P. (1984). *The situational leader.* Escondido, CA: Center For Leadership Studies.

Hersey, P., & Blanchard, K. H. (1969). *Management of organizational behavior: Utilizing human resources.* Englewood Cliffs, NJ: Prentice Hall.

House, R. M., & Hayes, R. L. (2002). School counselors: Becoming key players in school reform. *Professional School Counseling, 5*, 249–256.

Keys, S. G. (2000). Living the collaborative role: Voices from the field. *Professional School Counseling, 3*, 332–338.

Kouzes, J. M., & Posner, B. Z. (1995). *The leadership challenge.* San Francisco: Jossey-Bass.

Maslow, A. H. (1968). *Toward a psychology of being* (2nd ed.). Princeton, NJ: Van Nostrand.

Northouse, P. G. (2004). *Leadership: Theory and practice.* Thousand Oaks, CA: Sage Publications.

Rogers, C. (1980). A theory of therapy, personality, and interpersonal relationships as developed in the client-centered framework. In S. Koch (Ed.), *Psychology: A study of science, formulations of the person and the social context* (Vol. 3, pp. 184–256). New York: McGraw-Hill. (Original work published 1959)

Rogers, C. (1980). *A way of being.* Boston: Houghton Mifflin.

Rowley, W. J., Sink, C. A., & MacDonald, G. (2002). An experiential and systemic approach to encourage collaboration and community building. *Professional School Counseling, 3*, 298–307.

Senge, P. (1990). *The fifth discipline: The art and practice of the learning organization.* New York: Doubleday.

Sergiovanni, T. J. (1992). *Moral leadership: Getting to the heart of school improvement.* San Francisco: Jossey-Bass.

Sergiovanni, T. J. (1994). *Building community in schools.* San Francisco: Jossey-Bass.

Sergiovanni, T. J. (2001). *The principalship.* Boston: Allyn and Bacon.

CHAPTER 5
Leadership Style Exploration

REFLECTIONS OF A COUNSELOR LEADER

Joan was in her second year of a leadership position. She was the coordinator of the elementary school counseling program in her district. She spent most of her time supporting the elementary school counselors in various ways, writing required reports, attending district counseling meetings, arranging professional development presentations, and facilitating elementary school counseling meetings.

Joan had her own thoughts about the leadership roles that counselors can play in a school setting. She felt that school counselors played a vital role in developing and maintaining the overall school climate. Although Joan took a risk in challenging herself to become a more effective leader, she did not feel she had the knowledge of leadership practices that would help her. She had visions for the counseling program she coordinated, but was unsure of how to proceed. Joan felt that she was good at tweaking and refining the present counseling program but knew a time would come when someone would need to move the program forward strategically to keep up with the changing times and help families and school communities meet challenges. "I am not trained in leadership. I am a counselor."

Early in her career as a school counselor, Joan was reluctant to assume any position of leadership. She felt she did not have the knowledge base or training. She was at her first school appointment for a while before she felt comfortable enough to take a risk and assume a leadership role. When she did step up, she felt totally unprepared. "I felt definitely out of my element." She was concerned that she did not have the skills to be "assertive" and, therefore, was not prepared to be as strong an advocate as she wanted to be. In spite of her concern, Joan continued to avail herself of opportunities and challenges for leadership. She chaired committees, organized events, and participated in program development for systems change in her district.

Joan eventually felt she had made progress in developing into a strong leader and effective advocate. However, she still had doubts about her leadership ability and could not clearly articulate her leadership style. She described a recent crisis team meeting that she conducted to examine issues and resolve problems plaguing the crisis team and expressed her role in this way: "I thought of myself as more of a facilitator."

Case Discussion

Questions About This Case

- What were some of the key issues that Joan needed to address?
- What options might she have considered to strengthen her leadership ability as well as her confidence in that ability?
- What might be some ways for a school counselor to foster his/her own leadership development?
- What messages about school counselor roles and priorities does this scenario convey?
- What can we learn from this case example about leadership opportunities for school counselors?

Further Thoughts on This Case

Joan's story is similar to that of many school counselors in today's schools. Basic knowledge about leadership has not traditionally been treated as a major focus in school counseling preparation programs (Baker & Gerler, 2004). Yet more and more counselors in schools are being called upon to serve as leaders and advocates for all students. Joan's story provides a glimpse of what many of these counselors are feeling. Like Joan, many counselors are ready and willing to serve as leaders but some do so with trepidation and self-doubt. Some knowledge of leadership theory, style development, and awareness of their leadership capabilities would build the foundation for them to move forward with confidence.

CHAPTER OBJECTIVES

The objectives in this chapter are to:

1. Introduce leadership styles and encourage school counselors-in-training to consider their own leadership-style preferences.
2. Address the question of whether leaders are born or developed.

FROM LEADERSHIP THEORY TO LEADERSHIP STYLE

According to Northouse (2004), leadership style is the behavior pattern of someone who has influence over others. In this chapter we begin to look at leadership styles and the theories behind particular styles of leadership. Effective leaders should have a clear understanding of the leadership theories they subscribe to and feel confident that their style of leadership reflects the tenets of their preferred theory. This then manifests itself in behavior and practice. How do counselors know what their particular style of leadership is? Even if they have an idea, they may have difficulty recognizing and articulating their style to others. When asked, most will say something like, "I believe in participatory management." Or "I have an open-door policy." This chapter is designed to help counselors explore various styles of leadership that follow from the theories reviewed in Chapter 4 and to see the value in assessments that guide them to understanding and feeling comfortable with leadership. Such understanding and sense of comfort allows school counselors to become confident in the roles of leader, advocate, and collaborator.

It is important to remember to allow yourself to enjoy the process. It is not unusual to have been programmed to believe that an emerging leader needs to practice a style he/she admires or that one style is more "correct" than another. Learning to appreciate and trust that one's belief system and core values will direct one to the theory and style that fits best will contribute to the enjoyment of discovery as one begins to recognize and accept his/her leadership style. Bennis (1989) shared his view of leader development:

> No leader sets out to be a leader. People set out to live their lives expressing themselves fully. When that expression is of value, they become leaders. So the point is not to become a leader. The point is to become yourself, to use yourself completely—all your skills, gifts and energies—in order to make your vision manifest. You must withhold nothing. You must, in sum, become the person you started out to be, and to enjoy the process of becoming (p. 111).

Chapter 4 included a review of relevant educational leadership theory and models for counselors. In order to provide some understanding of moving from theory to practice, this chapter creates a bridge from theory to the reality of a leadership style.

In his book *Practicing the Art of Leadership,* Green (2001) provides an in-depth review of leadership theory and leadership practices. He focuses on school leadership and reviews the early studies on leadership behavior/styles, including the Iowa studies, the Ohio studies, and the Michigan studies. These three studies are summarized in the following sections.

The Iowa Studies

Green examined the literature on the Iowa studies by citing Lewin, Lippett, and White (1939). These studies, conducted by researchers at the University of Iowa, identified leaders practicing three basic behavioral styles: autocratic, democratic, and laissez-faire (Green, 2001). They found autocratic leaders to be direct, in charge, and nonparticipative in shared decision-making practices. Democratic leaders were more participative and more inclined to share decision-making practices. Laissez-faire leaders were more inclined to just allow things to happen with little involvement or concern.

The Autocratic Style

The autocratic leadership style does not allow for input or feedback from others. This approach sees others as followers only. Decisions, policies, and rules of the environment are made with the expectation that the leader knows best. An autocratic leader is not a team or participative type of leader. In fact, he/she expects to direct and handle all projects and has difficulty delegating to others. The autocratic style does not fare well with a committee structure. This leadership style may seem negative to some; however, in many situations the autocratic leadership style is more comforting for subordinates, who see the leader as very knowledgeable and decisive.

The Democratic Style

The democratic leader delights in participation and group thinking. Democratic leaders are comfortable with team efforts and empower others. They enjoy environments where relationship building is a priority. This leadership style may seem ideal to some; however, sometimes a more direct approach may be necessary, and democratic leaders may seem weak, indecisive, and incapable of thinking independently.

The Laissez-Faire Style

The laissez-faire leadership style allows others with confidence and expertise to move forward without the leader's input or assistance. Laissez-faire leaders provide little leadership or direction to others. They work well with competent and knowledgeable persons. Sometimes, however, a less-able group may flounder on its own because of lack of leadership.

The leadership theory most relevant to the styles observed in the Iowa studies is the Situational Leadership Theory. In the Situational Leadership approach, the leader must assess the situation, the task, and/or the environment to determine which style would be most effective.

The Three Leadership Styles in Practice

The Greenberg Unified School District has been informed that state test scores indicate that three schools in the district—Oakdale, Marshall, and Riverview—have been declared "underperforming" elementary schools. The superintendent has been informed by the state superintendent's office that if the schools do not show marked improvement by the next testing period, the state will take over these schools. The superintendent has charged each of the principals with the task of improving test scores in their schools, but they must decide what to do and what resources they will need. The following is an example of how leaders with different leadership styles tackled this task.

Oakdale School: The Autocratic Style   Mr. Nelson had been a school principal for fifteen years. He had been principal at Oakdale for five years. He knew the community well, and although he had an experienced faculty and staff, he knew they looked to him for leadership and guidance. Mr. Nelson felt that he must come up with a plan to benefit the students and keep up the morale of the teachers and staff. Mr. Nelson decided that an after-school tutoring program would be the best solution. He would find money in his school budget to pay tutors and ask the teachers to identify those students who would benefit the most from tutoring services.

Marshall School: The Laissez-Faire Style   Ms. Washington was the principal of Marshall School for over twenty years. She saw a lot of change in the neighborhood and the students of today compared to the students of twenty years ago. She felt that she had an experienced faculty with the best interests of all the students in their hearts. She decided that each teacher knew best how to provide lessons that would increase the test scores of their students. Ms. Washington decided to present the problem to the teachers and let them determine how best to increase the test scores of the students in their classrooms.

Riverview School: The Democratic Style   Ms. Otero was in her second year as a school administrator. She was disappointed by the test score results. She felt the faculty and staff had put much effort into improving the academic achievement of the students. She knew that the thought of the state taking over the school would cause the morale of both faculty and staff to plummet. Because the impact of the decisions she would make would affect the entire Riverview School community, Ms. Otero felt that all stakeholders involved should play a part in deciding how to improve student achievement by the next testing period. She knew that time was of the essence so she immediately began to plan strategies for a democratic process of resolving issues for improving student achievement at the school.

Comparing the Three Principals' Styles

Each of the principals decided to use a particular style based on his/her comfort zone and the readiness of the community involved. Mr. Nelson, the principal of Oakdale School, knew his faculty and staff well enough to know that they expected him to provide the solution. Their thinking was "You are the leader in charge. Tell us what to do, and we will do it." Ms. Washington, the principal of Marshall School, knew that she had an experienced faculty who put every effort into improving student achievement. Her solution was to provide resources and support and to allow the teachers to decide how they wanted to work with students and families to resolve issues causing poor academic achievement. Their thinking was "We are the experts. We know our students. We will attend to the problem. Please don't get in our way."

Ms. Otero, the principal of Riverview School, decided that everyone involved should have a part in developing strategies for improving student achievement. She felt that the entire school community had a stake in what happened at their school and the success of the students. She felt that a democratic process was important, where all involved will have opportunities for input in resolving issues of student achievement. Miss Otero decided that in her community a democratic solution would be more effective and more likely to succeed.

Self-Assessment and Exploration

This exercise involves matching leadership styles with situations.

Instructions: Read the following descriptions of school situations. Identify the leadership style you determine to be the most appropriate for each situation. Record the style you chose and your rationale in the space provided. Meet with a small group of four to five members and share your responses and rationale. The group should come to a consensus on the best style for each situation. Select one group member to report group decisions to the larger group. After all groups have reported, compare and discuss the rationales of each group's decisions.

1. The school office manager answers the phone and hears a raspy voice stating that there is a bomb in the school. She immediately reports this to the principal.

    Leadership Style: _____

    Rationale: _____

    _____

    _____

2. School attendance has dropped to 92 percent. In this state, if a school does not have an average annual attendance rate of 94 percent, it is declared an underperforming school regardless of test scores, and the state has the option of taking over the management of the school.

    Leadership Style: _____

    Rationale: _____

    _____

    _____

3. Morale at the school has reached an all-time low. Students are underperforming academically. Discipline problems are increasing. Teachers are unwilling to commit any time outside of their contract hours. Very few parents are involved in the school.

    Leadership Style: _____

    Rationale: _____

    _____

    _____

4. The school has received a substantial donation, with a stipulation that the funds be used to reward school employees.

    Leadership Style: _____

    Rationale: _____

    _____

    _____

5. Students have been reporting an increasing number of bullying incidents on the playground, in the bathrooms, in the lunchroom, and on the way home.

    Leadership Style: _____

Rationale: _____

_____

_____

The Ohio Studies

In a review of the Ohio studies, Green (2001) reported on the work of Hemphill and Coons (1997/1957) and Stogdill & Coons (1997), who designed a questionnaire that identified perceived behaviors of effective leaders. The Leadership Behavior Description Questionnaire (LBDQ) asked individuals to rate the behavior of their supervisors and was administered to hundreds of individuals in education, the military, and industrial settings (Northouse, 2004). The results of the analysis of this questionnaire placed leadership behavior in two categories: task-oriented leadership behavior and people-oriented leadership behavior. Task-oriented leaders were more inclined to pay attention to *structure*: schedules, performance, and deadlines. People-oriented leaders leaned more toward *consideration concerns*: the well-being of others, building trust, and including others in the decision-making process.

The results of the Ohio studies contributed to a model of leadership behavior that formed four quadrants.

Quadrant 1: High Consideration/Low Structure
Quadrant 2: High Structure/High Consideration
Quadrant 3: Low Structure/Low Consideration
Quadrant 4: High Structure/Low Consideration

Northouse (2004) discusses the Ohio studies in a chapter titled "Style Approach" and states that these behaviors are essentially what leaders do: provide structure and nurture. According to Northouse, a major task for researchers has been to determine when and how a leader mixes task and relationship behaviors to be the most effective in a given situation.

Whereas the Iowa studies addressed three styles of leadership, the Ohio studies focused on a model of leadership behavior that identified four styles of leadership: Servant Leadership, Empowered Leadership, Moral Leadership, and Situational Leadership. These are the theories that most likely encompass the leadership styles in each of the four quadrants. In each of these theories, providing structure is a vital part of the leader's responsibility. Fostering and nurturing the success and development of the individual is an important factor in the leader's effectiveness.

The Michigan Studies

The Michigan studies identified two types of leadership behaviors: Employee Orientation and Production Orientation. Employee Orientation is a style of behavior with a strong human relations emphasis. Personal needs and individuality are valued. Production Orientation values the structure that contributes to the accomplishment of the task. These styles of behavior are similar to the behaviors found in the Ohio research. Employee Orientation is similar to Consideration, and Production Orientation is similar to Initiating Structure. Theories relevant to the Michigan studies are similar to those cited for the Ohio studies: Servant Leadership, Empowered Leadership, Moral Leadership, and Situational Leadership. The human relations emphasis involves the concepts of servant and moral leadership. The style emphasizing structure for the completion of the task requires the ability to delegate and arrange for success as emphasized in empowerment and situational leadership.

THE STYLE APPROACH TO SCHOOL COUNSELOR LEADERSHIP

School counselors are now being asked to lead the charge for systemic change in the areas of social justice, equity, and school achievement. What would be a good style of leadership for a school counselor when developing a plan of action in these areas? It is worthwhile to reflect upon one's leadership style. School counselors should consider whether they prefer a style concerned with structure and task. It may be important to a school counselor to focus on the task at hand and the organizational structure that will contribute to its completion in a timely manner. Another counselor's style may be to focus on the technical and production aspects of a job (as described in the Michigan studies) and the task behaviors such as organizing the work activities and defining role responsibilities (described in the Ohio studies as Initiating Structure). Or, still another counselor's style may lean more toward the behaviors identified in the Ohio studies, such as consideration. This style focused on developing trust and building relationships. Research indicates that each style can be effective depending on the situation. Northouse commented on the style approach to leadership.

> The style approach broadened the scope of leadership research to include the behavior of leaders and what they do in various situations. No longer was the focus of leadership on the personal characteristics of leaders; it was expanded to include what leaders did and how they acted (Northouse, 1997, p. 41).

Early research studies cited in Northouse (2004) and Green (2001, 2005) indicate that styles of leadership fall into two categories: Task-oriented behavior or relationship-oriented behavior. Some situations require task behavior and some situations require supportive behavior by the leader. It is helpful to know your preference for a style behavior and to know when to adjust your style for a given situation.

Numerous leadership theories have evolved on the study of leadership and leadership behaviors. These studies have helped clarify the importance of the role of leaders in ensuring the success of organizations and those who make the organizations work. School counselors are being called upon to play a vital leadership role in schools and current school-reform movements. This requires that school counselors employ individual leadership and advocacy strategies and then move from an individual focus to a systemic focus (National Center for Transforming School Counseling, the Education Trust, 2003). Counselors need to recognize their leadership style and understand how to merge their style with those of other leaders who are playing major roles in developing policies and wrestling with issues prominent in school-reform efforts. A brief look at the research on leadership theories and the style approach to leadership can be useful in moving toward this goal.

Core Values and Leadership Styles

Our core values guide us in determining our behavior and practices. Knowing, understanding, and appreciating our core values helps give us confidence to step out of the box of expected behavior and act as a catalyst for behavior that is right and necessary in difficult situations. This is what separates a leader from a nonleader. One way counselors can start to analyze their deep-rooted core values during counselor training is to reflect upon the answers to the following questions:

1. What do I appreciate most about my character?
2. What would I most like to change about my character?
3. What principles do I believe in?
4. What assumptions do I live by?

Reflecting upon these four questions is a basic start to analyzing deep fundamental values and to clarifying some basic understandings about one's character.

The next step is to interpret how the answers to these questions manifest themselves in terms of how a school counselor wants to be in life, what the counselor wants to do in life, and how he/she wants to behave in life situations. Some other questions to ponder might be the following: Do my core values allow me to treat others as I would like to be treated? Do my core values allow me to do the "right" thing when making difficult decisions that might affect the livelihood of others? Do my core values allow me to be the person I really want to be? Exploring core values will help you understand why you may be more comfortable with one leadership style over another as a school counselor.

As the research on styles and theories of leadership demonstrates, there may be times when one style would be more effective than another, depending on the situation, the organizational structure of the environment, or the people involved. Knowing one's preferred style of leadership will let the counselor know whether that style or another style is likely to be most effective in a given situation, or even whether it might be most prudent to remove oneself from the environment and the situation all together.

Chapter 4 presented concepts from Covey (1991), who discusses core values and the development of a personal and professional mission statement. In his book *Principle-Centered Leadership* (1991), he devotes a chapter to the development of what he terms a *universal mission statement*. Covey focuses on the self-development of managers and leaders of organizations as they learn key principles of leading from within. He addresses the development of the mission statement:

> It attempts to encompass, in one brief sentence, the core values of the organization; it creates a context that gives meaning, direction, and coherence to everything else. To be functional, mission statements should be short so that people can memorize and internalize them. But they also need to be comprehensive (pp. 295–296).

If core values guide leadership behavior, the mission statement based on those core values creates direction and cements the commitment to stand by and practice those values. The school counselor as educational leader finds inspiration, direction, and continuing commitment in regularly reviewing and internalizing his/her mission statement.

Are Leaders Born or Developed?

We have attempted to make the argument that core values guide leadership behavior. Core values develop from our cultural practices, family traditions, and life experiences. If this argument holds true, then we all have leadership capabilities. It is how we develop and strengthen those capabilities that makes us the leader we choose to be. It is our leadership practices that determine whether we are effective or ineffective leaders in our environment. The first step is to understand our own preferred style of leadership and appreciate the research studies that clarify leadership styles for us. The next step is to make the commitment to live by our principles and values and to broaden the knowledge base and develop the skills to best apply our leadership capabilities.

CHAPTER SUMMARY

A school counselor's leadership style transfers to his/her behavior and practices. Having an understanding of leadership styles is an important component of one's leadership development. When aspiring leaders know the leadership theory that aligns with their style of leadership, they are likely to demonstrate more confidence in their interactions with others and in their decision-making practices. Research indicates that one particular style of leadership is not appropriate in all situations. School counselor educational leaders who are aware of various leadership styles can determine how they will respond to different environments, situations, and problem-solving opportunities.

Self-assessments and explorations of core values can assist school counselors in recognizing their individual leadership styles. Through reflection on deep fundamental values, the counselor leader develops a map for character development and change where indicated. It is often said that everyone has leadership capabilities. It is how we develop and strengthen these capabilities that determine the type of leader we will be. Developing a mission statement and setting goals for how to accomplish the mission is a hallmark of leadership behavior.

REVIEW AND REFLECT

1. What leadership theory do you prefer? Why? Reflect upon the theories presented in this book or other theories of leadership you have studied. Discuss with a partner and present an example of the behavior of a leader implementing this theory effectively.

    _____

    _____

    _____

    _____

    _____

_____

_____

_____

2. Write a position paper expressing your opinion regarding the question, "Are leaders born or developed?" In a large group, use a chalk- or whiteboard or a large sheet of paper to contribute to one or both of two lists with the following headings: 1. Why I think leaders are born 2. Why I think leaders are developed. Follow with a group discussion about the strongest points for each position.
3. Divide into groups of three. Each member of the group will play a different leadership-style role: autocratic, democratic, and laissez-faire. The scenario for the leader is that referrals to the office have increased dramatically in the past month. You are not sure what is causing the problem with behavior. Approach the problem according to the style assigned. Follow with small-group discussions of the advantages and disadvantages of each style in the given scenario. Report key findings to your larger group.

RELEVANT WEBSITES

American Association of School Administrators: www.aasa.org/
American School Counselor Association: www.schoolcounselor.org
Association for Supervision and Curriculum Development: www.ascd.org
Eye on Education: www.eyeoneducation.com
National Association of Secondary School Principals:
    www.principals.org/www.questia.com/
Reviews of educational policies and practices effective in closing the achievement
    gap: www.ed.gov/databases/ERIC_Digests/ed460191.html
The Education Trust: www.edtrust.org
The International Center for Leadership in Education: www.daggett.com/
The School Leadership Development Unit: www.sofweb.vic.edu.au/pd/schlead/
    http://21stcenturyschools.northcarolina.edu/center

REFERENCES

Baker, S. B., & Gerler, E. R., Jr. (2004). *School counseling for the twenty-first century*. Upper Saddle River, NJ: Pearson Education.

Bennis, W. (1989). *On becoming a leader*. Cambridge, MA: Perseus Books.

Covey, S. R. (1991). *Principle-centered leadership*. New York: Simon & Schuster.

Education Trust. (2003). *Transforming school counseling initiative* [Brochure]. Washington, DC: Author.

Green, R. L. (2001). *Practicing the art of leadership*. Upper Saddle River, NJ: Merrill Prentice Hall.

Hemphill, J. K., & Coons, A. E. (1997). *Development of the leader behavior description questionnaire*. In R. M. Stogdill & A. E. Coons (Eds.) *Leader behavior: Its description and measurement*. Columbus: Ohio State University, Bureau of Business Research.

Hersey, P. (1984). *The situational leader*. Escondido, CA: Center for Leadership Studies.

Hersey, P., & Blanchard, K. (1969). Life-cycle theory of leadership. *Training and Development Journal, 23,* 26–34.

Kouzes, J. M., & Posner, B. Z. (1995). *The leadership challenge.* San Francisco: Jossey-Bass.

Lewin, K., Lippitt, R., & White, R. K. (1939). Patterns of aggressive behavior in experimentally created "social climates." *Journal of Science Psychology, 10,* 271–299.

MacGregor, B. (1978). *Leadership.* New York: Harper & Row.

Northouse, P. G. (2004). *Leadership theory and practice.* Thousands Oaks, CA: Sage Publications.

Sergiovanni, T. J. (1992). *Moral leadership.* San Francisco: Jossey-Bass.

Stogdill, R. M., & Coons, A. E. (Eds.) (1997). *Leader behavior: Its description and measurement.* Columbus: Ohio State University, Bureau of Business Research.

CHAPTER 6
Leadership Assessment

AN EXPLORATION OF A LEADER'S POTENTIAL

Jamie had been a school counselor at the middle school level for five and a half years. During her years as a professional school counselor, she shared the belief with the other counselors on her team that the school counselors were there primarily for the students and the teachers. She was unsure about what type of relationship she should have with the administration and wondered if it would be possible someday to serve as a member of an educational leadership team with members of the administration.

She had the opportunity to attend the American School Counselor Association national conference for two consecutive years and had seen presentations on the new vision for school counseling. This vision included the role of school counselor as educational leader who advocates for all students and for systemic change. With encouragement from the district guidance coordinator, she had begun to lead the counselors in her department toward aligning their school counseling program with the National Model. She enjoyed taking on this leadership role and began to think about what leadership skills she had and how she could further develop her leadership potential to contribute even more effectively.

Case Discussion

Questions About This Case

- What were some of the key questions about leadership considered by this school counselor?

- What options might she have explored to address questions about working with members of the administration and about developing her own leadership potential?
- What might be some ways to foster leadership knowledge and skills while working as a school counselor?
- What messages about school counselor roles and priorities does this scenario convey?
- What can we learn from this case example about working with other personnel in a school?

Further Thoughts on This Case

Jamie realized that she needed some direction to assess her leadership potential. She spoke with the district guidance coordinator, who recommended that she attend the state counselors' leadership academy. She applied to the district and obtained approval and funding for the academy. She anticipated that the academy would build her confidence as an educational leader and strengthen her resolve to accept the challenge to become a new-vision school counselor.

In the initial session of the academy Jamie learned that one place to start is with self-awareness, which one can gain through various self-assessments. Throughout the academy experience she learned a considerable amount about educational leadership and her own leadership style, and she left with a concrete plan for leadership self-improvement. In addition, Jamie had identified a mentor who could coach her in successful achievement of her leadership-improvement goals and objectives.

CHAPTER OBJECTIVES

In Chapter 5 we introduced the idea that we can develop our leadership capabilities. To understand how to do this, it helps to evaluate ourselves to determine which of our capabilities need to be developed and strengthened. Self-assessments allow us to do this. Sometimes self-assessments can affirm attributes we were aware of but had never acknowledged as a strength to be applied in a meaningful way. Sometimes self-assessments can help us understand the capabilities we have to develop or strengthen. Finally, self-assessments can help us recognize those areas which call for change. This knowledge, if we act on it wisely, can build the confidence we need to accept the risk of new leadership opportunities. It is up to the counselor trainee to decide how to use the results of such assessments in planning future development.

The main objectives of this chapter are to:

1. Identify and describe appropriate leadership assessments for school counselors.
2. Discuss elements of self-assessments and self-assessment devices.
3. Provide a framework for the understanding of leadership assessment results.

ELEMENTS OF SELF-ASSESSMENT

Self-assessments present a glimpse of respondents in the area of the trait being assessed. For example, an assessment of behavioral characteristics can help respondents see their particular behavior compared with other types of behavior in the same environment or circumstance. In an assessment of personality characteristics, respondents can receive feedback about their particular personality characteristics as compared with others.

Self-Assessment Devices

Self-assessment devices are usually in the form of questions carefully crafted in order to allow respondents to answer easily and without the need for extensive reflection. They usually have a very low level of risk. Their worth depends on whether respondents are introspective and honest (Miles & Miles, 1982, unpublished). Some self-assessment devices ask the respondent to respond to a word, statement, or picture. Responses are analyzed and scored to provide the feedback to the respondent. The most effective devices have undergone formal reliability and validity analyses with extensive research of pertinent theories.

Many self-assessment devices are used as training tools and may not have gone through formal reliability and validity analyses but rely instead on the feedback of trainers and various other sources. There are many self-assessment devices on the market. Some are referred to as surveys, inventories, or personality tests and are designed to help respondents find out more about themselves. Instruments include self-assessments of various types of skills, management and leadership styles, and personality characteristics. There are self-assessments to guide career choices and assess job satisfaction. Some assessments are timed, and range from ten to forty-five minutes or longer in duration. Others do not have an established time limit. The next section presents and recommends some assessments for school counselors who want to explore and understand more about themselves and others in preparation for stronger leadership and advocacy roles.

The Myers-Briggs Type Indicator

The Myers-Briggs Type Indicator® (MBTI) provides a framework for understanding human behavior (Myers, McCaulley, Quenk, & Hammer, 2003). It is introduced in this chapter for counselors because it purports to help individuals understand their own behavior, thoughts, and feelings. This assessment helps people identify their strengths and weaknesses. It helps them understand themselves, their motivations, and potential areas for professional growth (DeVoss & Andrews, 2003). The MBTI is a self-report questionnaire based on Carl Jung's theory that behavior is predictable. According to Myers, McCaulley, Quenk, and Hammer (2003), Jung's theory generated a framework within which individual characteristics are related to individual preferences. There are sixteen psychological types based on Jung's theory.

Isabel Myers and Katharine Briggs developed the Myers-Briggs Type Indicator, the original purpose of which was to assist people in understanding and recognizing their skills and interests in various careers. Years of research went into the development of the MBTI, and it is widely used now in organizations as a tool for communication practices, decision making, team building, and overall leadership development of their employees. The MBTI is also a useful tool for leadership development for educational leaders.

The MBTI assesses psychological types along four dimensions, or preferences: Extraversion–Introversion, Sensing–Intuiting, Thinking–Feeling, and Judging–

Perceiving. The first dimension, Extraversion–Introversion, does not refer to gregariousness or shyness but identifies where people get their energy (McAlpine, Segal, & Hartzler, 1994). Those who prefer Extraversion usually focus outwardly on people, things, and actions. They are energized by being with others, take the initiative when making contact with others, and prefer to talk to sort out thoughts and feelings. Those who prefer Introversion need time alone, do their best when allowed to internalize, reflect before acting, and allow others to initiate contact.

The second preference dimension, Sensing–Intuiting, describes how people attend to and take in data. People who prefer Sensing are usually methodical, adamant about details, and focused on the here and now, whereas those who prefer Intuiting are imaginative, unconventional, and intellectual, with a mental focus on the future.

The third preference dimension, Thinking–Feeling, describes how people process data and make decisions through Thinking or Feeling. People who prefer Thinking tend to be critical, logical, and questioning. They make decisions objectively and impersonally, while considering the causes of events and where the decisions might lead. They value consistency and equality over harmony and rely on logic and principles. On the other hand, people who prefer Feeling make decisions subjectively and personally, weighing values and choices and how they matter to others. They are seen by others as fair-minded and are apt to seek consensus.

The fourth preference dimension, Judging–Perceiving, concerns the way we organize the outer world. People who prefer Judging set priorities, anticipate schedules, and know when they are finished with a project or task. They value order and structure and prefer a planned approach. People who prefer Perceiving like to have options, value flexibility, and easily tolerate ambiguity. They enjoy complexity and remain open for more information before finishing a task or project. They generally enjoy the process of doing and looking at all the possibilities. They are energized by last-minute rushes and enjoy surprises.

Each of these preference dimensions is represented by a letter—Extraversion-E, Introversion-I, Sensing-S, Intuiting-N, Thinking-T, Feeling-F, Judging-J, Perceiving-P. Respondents are asked to select the letter representing their preference on one side of each of the four preference scales, thus selecting the four letters that make up their self-selected type. There are sixteen possible types (see Table 6-1).

It is most beneficial to do this self-assessment with a trained facilitator, who can score the instrument and provide a knowledgeable interpretation of one's individual

Table 6-1   Type Table

ISTJ	ISFJ	INFJ	INTJ
ISTP	ISFP	INFP	INTP
ESTP	ESFP	ENFP	ENTP
ESTJ	ESFJ	ENFJ	ENTJ

From Consulting Psychologist Press, Inc.

personality type. For example, the following excerpt is part of the type description of ISTJ (Introversion/Sensing/Thinking/Judging):

> ISTJs judge the information they take in logically, analytically, and impersonally. They approach things from a practical point of view. They want things to be functional. They have little interest in or tolerance for exotic or impractical ideas or schemes. They are modest and down-to-earth. They apply common sense to whatever they do. Few details get by them. They see the "fine print" perhaps better than any other type (Brownsword, 1990).

The authors of the MBTI are careful to point out that the individual preferences in our personalities do not operate alone, but rather there is synergism among the four preferences. The MBTI provides a means to improve self-understanding as well as to better understand and appreciate others. Its benefits also include improving communication skills with others whose preferences are different from our own and who can provide insight in team-building efforts. The MBTI is a popular self-assessment tool. Some university and community testing services offer it for a fee.

True Colors Self-Assessment System

Don Lowry is the creator and author of the True Colors concept: a "state of mind and a metaphor for understanding human characteristics and how intrinsic behavior must be differentially rewarded" (1990, p.1). The theory behind True Colors is based on Hippocrates' identification of four personality types (Sanguine, Choleric, Phlegmatic, and Melancholic); the work of Carl Jung, who theorized four psychological types (Intuition, Feeling, Body, and Intellect); the work of Katharine Briggs and Isabel Myers in the development of the MBTI personality type inventories; and David Keirsey's research on temperament theories and the development of the Keirsey Temperament Sorter.

True Colors is based on the assumption that different people react differently to their environment. This system assigns a color to each of the different personality types. The colors selected to represent the personality types have little to do with one's favorite color or the colors of one's clothes. Lowry (1990) selected the colors to reflect meaning related to the individual and his/her attitudes as he/she navigates through life. The four colors selected for this system are Blue, Gold, Green, and Orange.

Following is a brief description of some of the identifying behaviors of the various personality types:

Blue—harmonious, calm, sensitive, and empathetic, with the need to be authentic.
Green—perseverant, tenacious, and complex, with the need to be ingenious.
Orange—energetic, action-oriented, eager, and bold, with the need to be skillful.
Gold—responsible, loyal, practical, and punctual, with the need to be responsible.

The True Colors self-assessment device is administered through a system that has three components: character cards, word sort, and "edutainment." The assessment usually begins with character cards. Respondents are given cards with characters demonstrating behaviors associated with each of the colors. They must select the color card with the characters who are behaving most like them.

The word sort is another part of the system. Respondents are asked to select from groups of three words the group that best describes them. They are asked to score themselves to determine which groups of words fit them best. Each group of words has a value that, when added together, gives a numeric score. Having a high score for a particular color indicates that an individual most likely exhibits the personality characteristics identified with that color.

Lowry also uses entertainment in the system as another medium to convey the power and dynamics of the True Colors concept. Respondents are exposed to video shows or live vignettes of the different color characters demonstrating their behaviors as they interact with others. Lowry calls this part of the system "edutainment," and he believes that

> . . . the entertainment format breaks down resistance and allows everyone who experiences it to become aware of their own True Colors, which in turn leads them on the path of discovering themselves as a "True Colors Person" . . . one who is aware of who he or she is, who can adapt to others, and one who can take action for success in any context while preserving their own esteem and that of others (*True Colors Training Manual*, 1990).

Many school counselors are familiar with the language of True Colors and practice the True Colors concepts in their work with teachers and students. Counselors are aware of group dynamics and the interaction of different personality characteristics. School counselors use this awareness in helping their clientele interact positively with others (that is, teacher to student, student to student). However, school counselors can also use this knowledge and awareness to strengthen their leadership capabilities and help them begin to move into leadership and advocacy positions. As one practicing counselor stated in her presentation to counseling students at the practicum stage, "Everyone in counseling needs to brighten all of their colors" (Carmen Hernandez's presentation to Counseling Process class, 9/21/04). She spoke about the need for counselors to be more involved in leadership roles in the counseling professional associations as well as on committees and school-wide leadership teams at their respective schools. The True Colors approach allows individuals to expand their perspective in the context of working with others and to improve the quality of this interaction in various situations and environments.

Self-Assessment and Exploration

The purpose of this exercise is to describe yourself based on the True Colors assessment system and analyze your self-assessment in terms of its implications regarding your leadership style.

A. True Colors Word Sort (Adapted from True Colors Training Manual, 1990)

Instructions: In the grid below, words are grouped together in boxes, and the boxes are arranged in rows, four boxes to a row. Score the groups of words in each row by giving the group of words that *most* describes you a score of 4, the group of words that *second most* describes you a 3, the group of words that is the *second least* descriptive of you a score of 2, and the group of words that *least* describes you a score of 1. Write the score in the space provided in the bottom right corner of each box. Proceed from left to right, scoring the groups of words in each row before proceeding to the next row.

Example:

Active Opportunistic Spontaneous	Parental Traditional Responsible	Authentic Harmonious Compassionate	Versatile Inventive Competent
3	2	4	1

In the example above, the respondent decided that of the four groups of words in the row,

Authentic/Harmonious/Compassionate is *most* descriptive of her (score 4)
Active/Opportunistic/Spontaneous is the *second most* descriptive (score 3)
Parental/Traditional/Responsible is the *second least* descriptive (score 2)
Vesatile/Inventive/Competent is the *least* descriptive of her (score 1).

Active Opportunistic Spontaneous	Parental Traditional Responsible	Authentic Harmonious Compassionate	Versatile Inventive Competent
—	—	—	—
Competitive Impetuous Impactful	Practical Sensible Dependable	Unique Empathetic Communicative	Curious Conceptual Knowledgeable
—	—	—	—
Realistic Open-minded Adventuresome	Loyal Conservative Organized	Devoted Warm Poetic	Theoretical Seeking Ingenious
—	—	—	—
Daring Impulsive Fun	Concerned Procedural Cooperative	Tender Inspirational Dramatic	Determined Complex Composed
—	—	—	—
Exciting Courageous Skillful	Orderly Conventional Caring	Vivacious Affectionate Sympathetic	Philosophical Principled Rational
—	—	—	—

Orange _____	Gold _____	Blue _____	Green _____

Total your scores for each column and place the total in the box below each column. When you have finished, read the descriptions of the four color personality characteristics below.

Orange: I act on a moment's notice. I consider life as a game. I value skill, resourcefulness, and courage. I am a natural troubleshooter.

Gold: I need to follow rules and respect authority. I have a strong sense of what is wrong and right in life. I need to be useful and to belong. I am concrete and organized.

Blue: I look for meaning and significance in life. I need to contribute, to encourage, and to care. I value integrity and unity in relationships

Green: I seek knowledge and understanding. I live life by my own standards. I am a nonconformist, a visionary, and a problem solver.

B. Relating True Colors to Leadership

1. In small groups, discuss the strengths and pitfalls for leaders whose dominant characteristics fall into each of the four color categories.

Orange

Strengths for Leadership   Pitfalls for Leadership

_____   _____

_____   _____

_____   _____

Gold

Strengths for Leadership   Pitfalls for Leadership

_____   _____

_____   _____

_____   _____

Blue

Strengths for Leadership   Pitfalls for Leadership

_____   _____

_____   _____

_____   _____

Green

Strengths for Leadership   Pitfalls for Leadership

_____   _____

_____   _____

_____   _____

After determining your own True Colors, from most dominant to least dominant, and taking into consideration the related characteristics, write down what you think are the implications for you as a leader. Your notes will be useful as you complete a leadership improvement plan in Chapter 7.

Strengths for Leadership

_____

_____

_____

_____

_____

_____

_____

_____

_____

_____

Pitfalls for Leadership

_____

_____

_____

_____

_____

_____

_____

_____

_____

_____

Additional Self-Assessment

Leadership is not a mystical quality that only a select few are born with; it is a set of behaviors that both experienced and prospective leaders can use to turn challenging opportunities into remarkable success. Given the opportunity for feedback and practice, those who really want to lead can substantially improve their ability to do so (Kouzes & Posner, 2001).

THE LEADERSHIP PRACTICES INVENTORY

The Leadership Practices Inventory (LPI) is based on the research of James M. Kouzes and Barry Z. Posner, who have conducted research on leadership for more than eighteen years. Their conclusions are now based on more than 4,000 cases and 200,000 surveys, "because we wanted to provide up-to-date tools for training and learning about leadership" (Kouzes & Posner, 2001). Research results indicated a consistent pattern of leader behavior.

Five sets of behaviors became apparent and were referred to as five best practices in *The Leadership Challenge*, the book that reports this study (Kouzes & Posner, 1995). For each of the five best practices there are two strategies or commitments that provide counselors with a basis for learning to lead (DeVoss & Andrews, 2003). These five best practices became the foundation for a leadership model, which was briefly described in Chapter 4 of this book (Kouzes & Posner, 1995). In order to promote a more complete understanding of the Leadership Practices Inventory, additional information about this model, as presented in the *Leadership Practices Inventory Facilitator's Guide* (2001) is included here.

The first practice described in the model is Challenging the Process. The strategies or commitments involved in this practice are to search out opportunities to change, grow, innovate, and improve, and to experiment, take risks, and learn from accompanying mistakes. The premise of this practice is that leaders push others and themselves to exceed accepted limits.

The second practice is that of Inspiring a Shared Vision. The strategies or commitments for this practice involve envisioning an uplifting and ennobling future and enlisting others in a common vision by appealing to their values, interests, hopes, and dreams. The premise of this practice is that leaders believe they can make a difference. They have a vision for the future, believe in it, and work toward enlisting others to share that vision.

The third practice is Enabling Others to Act. Fostering collaboration by promoting cooperative goals and building trust is one of the strategies to implement this practice. A second strategy is to strengthen people by giving power away, providing choice, developing competencies, assigning critical tasks, and offering visible support. The premise of this practice is that leaders foster collaboration and build spirited teams.

The fourth practice is Modeling the Way. The strategies for this practice are to set an example by behaving in ways that are consistent with shared values and achieving small "wins" that promote consistent progress and build commitment. Leaders model ways to keep projects on course and break assignments down in order to achieve small successes along the way.

The fifth practice is Encouraging the Heart. This practice involves two commitments: recognizing individual contributions to the success of every project and celebrating team accomplishments. The premise of the fifth practice is that leaders know that members of a winning team need to share in the rewards of their effort. Leaders recognize the contributions that individuals make and employ a variety of ways (thank-you notes, public praise, smiles) to celebrate their efforts.

The Leadership Practices Inventory measures the leadership behaviors from this model. Administered in the form of a questionnaire, the LPI was developed to give managers feedback on how often they use best practices. The LPI-IC (Leadership Practices Inventory–Individual Contributor) was developed so that leaders who are not managers could get the same kind of feedback. It can be administered through the use of a self-report questionnaire and an observer's questionnaire, which is completed by a supervisor or several people who have observed the individual.

Empirical and statistical tests were conducted to determine the validity and reliability of the LPI-IC instruments. They found the questionnaires to be highly reliable in that the six statements for each practice are highly correlated. Test/retest reliability was high in that when someone takes and retakes the LPI-IC in a few months, without leadership training, the results are consistent. The instrument was found to have concurrent validity, face validity, and predictive validity. One can count on the results to predict behavior and to predict positive outcomes.

The Leadership Skills Inventory

During the 1980s, a group of educational administrators compiled a list of twelve essential leadership skills (Andrews & Schwanenberger, 2000). The National Association of Secondary School Principals (NASSP) Assessment Center used these skills as a basis for identifying potential leaders, and their work was reported in the *NASSP Bulletin* in September 1982. NASSP later revised this list and studies have shown that principals believe development of these skills will contribute to the success of individuals meeting the challenges of leadership in the 21st century (Andrews, 2000).

The Leadership Skills Inventory (Miles & Miles, 1982) asks respondents to rate their behavior in each of the following twelve essential leadership skills categories:

1. Problem Analysis — the ability to seek out relevant data and analyze complex information to determine the important elements of a problem situation, to search for information with a purpose.
2. Judgment — the ability to reach logical conclusions and make good decisions based on available information; skill in identifying needs and setting priorities; the ability to critically evaluate written communications.
3. Organizational Ability — the ability to plan, schedule, and control the work of others; skill in using resources in an optimal fashion; the ability to cope with a volume of paperwork and heavy demands on one's time.
4. Decisiveness — the ability to recognize when a decision is required and to act quickly.
5. Leadership — the ability to get others involved in solving problems; the ability to recognize when a group requires direction, to interact with a group effectively, and to guide the group to the accomplishment of a task.
6. Sensitivity — the ability to perceive the needs, concerns, and personal problems of others; skill in resolving conflicts; tact in working with people from different backgrounds; the ability to deal effectively with people concerning emotional issues; knowing what information to communicate and to whom.

7. Stress Tolerance — the ability to perform under pressure and with opposition; the ability to think on one's feet.

8. Oral Communication — the ability to make a clear oral presentation of facts and ideas.

9. Written Communication — the ability to express ideas clearly in writing and to write appropriately for different audiences.

10. Range of Interest — the competency to discuss a variety of subjects, for example, education, politics, current events, economics; the desire to actively participate in events.

11. Personal Motivation — the need to achieve in all activities attempted; recognition that work is important to personal satisfaction; the ability to be self-policing.

12. Educational Values — the possession of a well-reasoned philosophy; receptiveness to new ideas and change.

The profile inventory of each of the skills uses a Likert scale with a continuum starting with "always performing the skill in the way stated" to "never performing the skill in the way stated." The respondents are asked to rate their most current behavior.

Self-Assessment and Exploration

In this exercise, you will complete a Brief Miles Leadership Skills Inventory (adapted from Miles & Miles, 1982).

Instructions: For each of the items, circle the rating from 1 to 5 that indicates your typical behavior. On the scale provided, 1 indicates never displaying the behavior or characteristic, and 5 indicates always displaying the behavior or characteristic For example, in the Problem Analysis section, if you always examine all relevant sources of information, circle 5 as your response on that item. Remember, this is an inventory of your most current behavior. By assessing what you do presently, you can determine what skills you need to develop.

A. Problem Analysis	Never ⟵ ⟶ Always
1. I examine all relevant sources of information.	1 2 3 4 5
2. I establish criteria for judging the value of acquired data.	1 2 3 4 5
3. I establish criteria to help determine when the problem is solved.	1 2 3 4 5
4. I develop a list of the most pertinent issues that pertain to the problem.	1 2 3 4 5
5. I can eliminate the irrelevant issues that surround the problem.	1 2 3 4 5
Total Score:	_____

B. Judgment	
1. In making a judgment, I try first to determine who will be affected.	1 2 3 4 5
2. As I make decisions, I determine both long- and short-term impact.	1 2 3 4 5

3. I determine which criteria are most important in making a judgment.	1 2 3 4 5
4. I analyze the data surrounding an issue.	1 2 3 4 5
5. I refuse to alter a decision because of hearsay and imprecise data.	1 2 3 4 5

Total Score: _____

C. Organizational Ability

1. When I set priorities for myself, I consider time constraints.	1 2 3 4 5
2. When approaching a task, I consider its importance to others.	1 2 3 4 5
3. I develop clear plans of action.	1 2 3 4 5
4. I am willing to delegate tasks to those with needed skill and ability.	1 2 3 4 5
5. I have clear procedures for reporting and updating on tasks.	1 2 3 4 5

Total Score: _____

D. Decisiveness

1. I recognize when a decision is required by determining what the consequences will be if that decision is not made.	1 2 3 4 5
2. I list the alternatives to my decisions.	1 2 3 4 5
3. I make decisions in a timely fashion based upon available data.	1 2 3 4 5
4. I can resist pressure from others to change a decision too soon.	1 2 3 4 5
5. I establish criteria to test a decision.	1 2 3 4 5

Total Score: _____

E. Sensitivity

1. I try to elicit opinions about things that have an impact on others.	1 2 3 4 5
2. I work to reflect the point of view of others.	1 2 3 4 5
3. I seek feedback on my ability to accurately reflect others' views.	1 2 3 4 5
4. I try to consider implications of my action for all concerned.	1 2 3 4 5
5. I recognize that conflict may be a way of defining issues.	1 2 3 4 5

Total Score: _____

F. Oral Communication

1. I make clear oral presentations of facts and ideas.	1	2	3	4	5
2. I express myself clearly to a variety of audiences.	1	2	3	4	5
3. I use mannerisms of confidence.	1	2	3	4	5
4. I avoid using distractive mannerisms.	1	2	3	4	5
5. I have all presentational materials well organized.	1	2	3	4	5

Total Score: _____

Adapted from Mike Miles, PhD, and Ann A'Lee Miles, "Miles Leadership Skills Inventory." Copyright © 1982 by Miles & Miles. Reprinted by permission of Mike Miles, PhD, and Ann A'Lee Miles.

Review your score in each section. A score of 20 or higher in a section indicates that you have some strengths in that area of leadership. A score lower than 15 in a section indicates a weakness in that area of leadership. A score of 4 or 5 on a specific item indicates a strength on that particular behavior or characteristic. A score lower than 3 suggests a weakness on that behavior or characteristic.

Describe Your Strengths and Weaknesses

Identify and document your strengths and weaknesses for consideration in the leadership improvement plan you will develop in Chapter 7.

_____

_____

_____

_____

_____

_____

_____

_____

_____

_____

CHAPTER SUMMARY

When school counselors become aware of their strengths and weaknesses as leaders through self-assessment, they are better prepared to set their own performance objectives and choose outcome indicators for evaluating how they and the school counseling program in general contribute to the mission of the school. In addition, leadership self-assessments provide information to guide decisions about a school counselor's professional development needs. The self-assessment and appraisal processes can work together to foster continuous learning and self-improvement of the school counselor.

Self-assessments can be used as tools for self-improvement. This chapter has reviewed self-assessment devices that appear to be the most beneficial for school counselors who want to improve their leadership skills. The assessments not only provide feedback for leadership skills but also strengthen and affirm self-awareness. A greater self-awareness of who we are, where we gain our energies, and what behaviors we practice in our daily activities and interactions with others can build confidence for stepping up to the plate and taking on new challenges. For emerging leaders as well as experienced leaders, the feedback from self-assessments can assist in improving school counselors' abilities and expanding their capabilities.

REVIEW AND REFLECT

1. Write a letter to yourself that you will read five years from now congratulating yourself on all of your accomplishments. Make a list of the leadership skills and/or leadership behaviors you feel you would need to improve in order to accomplish your five-year goals. Include this letter in a leadership development journal you can use to document your progress.
2. Complete a leadership assessment. Based on the results, begin identifying your strengths and areas for improvement. Keep results and your notes available as you develop a leadership improvement plan using the format provided in Chapter 7. Note some ideas for goals and objectives. Ask a colleague to commit to observing your leadership behavior in the next few weeks. Plan to meet with your colleague two to three times in the next four to six months and ask for feedback on your progress.

RELEVANT WEBSITES

MBTI

Online Assessments: http://home.att.net/~personalassessments/online_assessments/mbti.html

CPP: http://www.cpp.com/products/mbti/index.asp

True Colors

True Colors: http://www.truecolors.org/

LPI

Corporate Library: www.corporatelibrary.org

REFERENCES

Andrews, M. F. (2000). *Skills for the twenty-first century educational leader.* Paper presented at the National Council of Professors of Educational Administration 54th Annual Summer Conference, Ypsilanti, MI.

Andrews, M. F., & Schwanenberger, M. (2000). The middle school principal and twelve essential leadership skills. Journal of the WRMLC: *The Middle Level Educator, 8(1),* 10–12.

Brownsword, A. W. (1990). *The type descriptions.* Nicasio, CA: HRM Press.

DeVoss, J. A., & Andrews, M. F. (2003). A new model for leadership and advocacy training in counselor education. *Arizona Counseling Journal, 23,* 7–13.

Kouzes, J. M., & Posner, B. Z. (1995). *The leadership challenge.* San Francisco: Jossey-Bass.

Kouzes, J. M., & Posner, B. Z. (2001). *Leadership practices inventory facilitator's guide.* San Diego, CA: Jossey-Bass/Pfeiffer.

Lowry, D. (1990). *True Colors training manual.* Corona, CA: True Colors.

McAlpine, R. W., Segal, M. L., & Hartzler, G. J. (1994). Script for an introductory MBTI group feedback (Version 1.0) [Computer software]. Gaithersberg, MD: Type Resources.

Miles, M., & Miles, A. (1982). *The leadership manual.* Unpublished manuscript.

Myers, I. B., McCaulley, M. H., Quenk, N. L., & Hammer, A. L. (2003). *MBTI manual: A guide to the development and use of the Myers-Briggs Type Indicator* (3rd ed.). Palo Alto, CA: CPP, Inc.

CHAPTER 7

The Leadership Improvement Plan

THE EXPERIENCED COUNSELOR LEADER

Bruce had worked at his present school for thirty-three years, serving as a school counselor for the past twelve years. There were three other counselors in the department and Bruce was the chair. In this position he held weekly meetings and provided direction for other counselors. Following is an abbreviated list of the duties and responsibilities of the high school counseling department chairperson in this school district:

1. Provides leadership of the school counseling department; serves as an advocate for all students; develops collaborative relationships; and works to create systemic change in the school that contributes towards academic success of all students.
2. Is responsible for the implementation of the district governing board approved Comprehensive Competency-Based Guidance Program (CCBG).
3. Represents the department at monthly district department meetings. Attends all monthly meetings.
4. Coordinates work of counselors in the department, counseling department secretary, and student aides assigned to the department.
5. Gathers statistical data on school counseling program, oversees completion of district and school required reports.
6. Coordinates, organizes, and distributes scholarship information.

7. Acts as a liaison between administration and the counseling department.
8. Coordinates all counseling department activities.
9. Prepares and facilitates the development of the yearly CCBG counselor agreements, counselors' calendar, and semester audits, and completes the semester audits for the department.
10. Facilitates weekly school counseling department meetings.
11. Attends weekly school department chairpersons' meetings and advisory council meetings.
12. Assists in and oversees the development of materials and plans for classroom visitation and registration orientation for students.
13. Coordinates ACT, SAT, PSAT, ASVAB, and AP testing.
14. Organizes materials and coordinates visits of colleges and technical schools.
15. Conducts orientation programs for incoming students.
16. Coordinates the operation of the Career Center.
17. Is responsible for organizing annual budget requests and ordering warehouse supplies.
18. Delegates responsibilities as appropriate, for example, peer counseling training and group organization.

When asked about his leadership style, Bruce responded that he felt he was a good listener, was nonthreatening, did things in a democratic way, and was well organized. He felt that because of the number of years he had been at this school, he was well integrated into the system and was a part of the leadership team. Although Bruce served as the department chairman he did not believe he was any more qualified than the other counselors in the department; he simply had been assigned different responsibilities. His belief was that "Good counselors had the skills already in them." He believed that core values determine your attitudes. "Some people are very smart but have a poor attitude. You can't teach people attitude."

Case Discussion

Questions About This Case

■ What were some of the key issues that this experienced school counselor in a changing school environment needed to address?
■ How closely do the responsibilities of the department chairman in this scenario align with the priorities for school counselors in the ASCA National Model?
■ How can a school guidance department effectively utilize the leadership skills of the department to support the mission of school counselors?
■ What messages about school counselor roles and priorities does this scenario convey?
■ What can we learn from this case example about working with other personnel in a school?

Further Thoughts on This Case

Bruce's story is a fast-forward for what may lie ahead for dedicated and courageous school counselors willing to meet the demands of a changing society. The long list of Bruce's responsibilities included developing collaborative relationships, creating systemic change when needed, and gathering and using statistical data for school improvement efforts to ensure student success. Bruce was a vital part of the leadership team, and in his words, "Provides input as to the pulse of what is happening on the campus." This type of leadership requires self-awareness and self-confidence. Knowing where one's abilities lie and knowing what and how to initiate plans for improvement is a necessity.

CHAPTER OBJECTIVES

Chapter 6 discussed self-assessments and how they can be useful in providing feedback for self-improvement. The results of self-assessments serve little purpose if they are not used to develop plans for improvement. It is also important to have an ongoing process of receiving continuous feedback from others, as well as strategies for self-monitoring and continued revisions of the leadership improvement plan when indicated.

The objectives of this chapter are to:

1. Provide a format for incorporating leadership assessment results into a leadership improvement plan.
2. Introduce a leadership improvement plan model that encompasses the essential elements of a good basic plan for individual improvement.

DEVELOPING A LEADERSHIP IMPROVEMENT PLAN

This model was originally developed for school administrators (Miles & Miles, 1982). It was called the Skill Development Plan and was used as a companion to the Leadership Behavior Profiles inventories (unpublished). It has since been revised to assist school counselors. The new version is intended to be used by anyone in his/her quest for leadership improvement.

Identify Areas for Improvement

The first stage of the leadership improvement model requires the respondent to analyze the data to determine the areas needing refinement. This leads to establishing the objectives of your plan. Self-assessment feedback provides a way to see when, how often, and how you practice a behavior or skill. Often the feedback is in the form of a numeric score or another indicator that gives value to an item or items on the assessment instrument or system. A careful analysis of this information will point to the areas of improvement you need to include in the objectives of your plan.

The Myers-Briggs Type Indicator provides information about particular personality types and provides insight into how a school counselor's type interacts with those with different personality types. In order to interact, lead, or negotiate with other personality types a school counselor's objective might be to find ways to develop a better understanding of another type or, as with the feedback from the Leadership Practices Inventory, to practice behaviors that inspire others. Careful analysis of the assessment chosen by the school counselor leader will identify areas for change or improvement. There may be several areas indicated. This model calls for the counselor to select one particular area in which to begin to implement strategies for improvement. The first step of this plan is identifying one area to address. Later, other areas can be added to the development plan.

Develop the Objectives of the Plan

Once the school counselor leader identifies the area to start with for leadership development, step 2 is to list the objectives for the plan. What specifically does the school counselor need to do to become more effective in the area selected for improvement? It is important to state objectives in specific terms. Let's use a specific example. Under the practice Enabling Others to Act in the Leadership Practices Inventory (Kouzes & Posner, 2001), the respondent rates certain behaviors. The rating of these behaviors indicates that the respondent never, rarely, sometimes, or often behaves in this way. If this is the area of concern the counselor chose to address, the objectives might be the same as those stated in the instrument:

Objective 1: Involve others in planning.
Objective 2: Treat others with respect.
Objective 3: Allow others to make decisions.
Objective 4: Develop cooperative relationships.

These would be listed as behaviors that need attention and would be stated in the form of objectives for this plan. Once the counselor has implemented this plan and achieved the objectives, he/she can select another area and formulate new objectives.

Select a Mentor

Step 3 is to select someone to serve as a mentor or coach. In selecting a mentor or coach for the plan, the school counselor will need to select someone who has successfully implemented or demonstrated the behaviors stated in the objectives. The counselor will need to discuss with that person the assessments that have highlighted the behavior he/she needs to work on and ask for assistance in implementing his/her plan for improvement.

Leaders need mentors who see in them what they don't recognize in themselves and challenge them to develop more fully. Effective leaders often credit their mentors for their challenging and empowering behaviors. It is worth the effort to search for and identify a good mentor who has desirable leadership qualities and the ability to facilitate the growth of their mentees. School counselors as educational leaders often have a diverse pool of prospective mentors within their working environment which may include other school counselors, administrators, and other school personnel.

Scheduling the dates and times for meetings is highly recommended. The frequency of meetings will depend on the mentor's and counselor's schedules; however, biweekly or -monthly meetings are suggested. The amount of time allotted for each meeting also depends on the busy schedule of two professional people. It is important to respect the availability of the mentor's as well as the counselor's time. Whatever time the mentor agrees to spend with the counselor should be planned and used well.

Searching for a Mentor

Begin looking for a mentor. Keep in mind that a mentor is a teacher, coach, and guide. Start by making a list of what you wish to gain from the mentoring relationship. List the qualities that you value in a mentor. Identify three people who have the qualities you seek in a mentor. Approach one of the three and arrange to meet with him/her to discuss the development of a mentoring relationship. Reflect on this process in your leadership development journal.

Valued Qualities in a Mentor	Mentoring Candidates
A.	1.
	2.
	3.
B.	1.
	2.
	3.
C.	1.
	2.
	3.
D.	1.
	2.
	3.
E.	1.
	2.
	3.

Develop Strategies to Address Objectives

Step 4 is probably the most important step after identifying the improvement needed. Carefully selected strategies will contribute to improvement. The mentor or coach can help craft behaviors to put into practice that will address the behavior identified for change. For the objective example cited in step 2, consider which behaviors one could put into practice that would indicate "treating others with respect." It would include allowing others to finish expressing their thoughts without interrupting. It would also include listening to others' ideas before insisting they listen to you first. This is where experienced mentors can share the things they do that make them effective in the area chosen for improvement.

The mentor and the counselor should develop an action plan for implementing the leadership development strategies. What will the counselor do? How often will the counselor do it? When should the counselor check to see how the strategy or strategies are working? There should be some discussion about how the school counselor will find opportunities or create opportunities to practice the strategies. Because the new behaviors are behaviors that counselors are probably not familiar or comfortable with, it is a good idea to make sure the selected behavior or practice is something the counselor really aspires to change. Implementing improvement strategies may take extensive effort. The mentor or coach can also support the counselor leader as he/she puts strategies into practice.

Develop Strategies to Monitor Progress

Step 5 is to develop strategies to monitor and check progress. First, the counselor should review the objectives and timelines developed in step 2. What are some steps the counselor can take to monitor the how, what, when, and where questions? Following are some recommended strategies to start this stage of the plan:

1. Keep a daily journal. Set aside the time to journal daily activities and interactions. You can do this at the end of the day or during the day as time permits. Describe the activities and interactions that occurred that day. Counselors should describe their type and level of involvement, for instance, whether they performed as leaders, participants, or observers or in some combination of roles and whether they were active or passive or a combination of both as they fulfilled their roles. They should also reflect on their behaviors and practices as they performed their duties and interacted with others. Counselors should consider whether they created or took advantage of opportunities to practice new behaviors. If so, what were their feelings? What was the impact on them or on others? Did they avoid practicing new behaviors? If so, they should ask themselves why. Counselors can learn a considerable amount from sharing the answers to these questions and their thoughts with their mentors the next time they meet. The mentor and school counselor may decide that things are moving along smoothly or see the need to make revisions to the plan.

2. The school counselor should solicit the aid of a trusted friend or colleague who has opportunities to observe the counselor in action. Counselors can share their plan with a friend or colleague as they did with their mentor. It is useful to ask the colleague or friend to make note of the counselor leader's behaviors as he/she puts the plan into practice. The counselor should ask the colleague to share his/her notes and observations. The counselor may benefit from encouraging the colleague to share his/her perception of how others viewed the counselor's behavior in a specific situation and what impact that behavior may have inspired in this situation or environment. This is a good time to simply listen and ask questions.

   Bolman and Deal (2002) indicate that asking others around us is the easiest way to get honest feedback. They postulate that it takes persistence and skill to frame the right questions. Initially, it may take some probing to get honest feedback. It may also require reassuring colleagues that one truly wants and values the feedback one is requesting of them. The feedback received from such observations and perceptions will provide much needed insight into how others view the counselor and how well the counselor is following through with his/her practice. Once again, discussing this feedback with the mentor may indicate a need to revise the development plan or may affirm the counselor leader's success in achieving his/her objectives.

3. Practice reflective exercises. "The heart of true leadership can only be found in the heart of the leader" (Bolman & Deal, 2001). In the book *Leading with Soul*, readers are taken on a spiritual journey of a leader in his search for "soul and spirit" and "depth and meaning" (Bolman & Deal, p. 4). Reflective thought was the driving force behind this search. Reflective practice provides the means for self-assessment and self-monitoring of our actions and behaviors. A school counselor may have asked, "What was I thinking?" at some time in his/her life. Actually, this is a very important question in reflective practice. What did I do and why did I handle a certain situation in the way that I did? Could I have behaved differently, and how will I react in this situation should it happen again? These are the kinds of questions school counselors should ask themselves during reflective practice. One can do reflective practice exercises at any time one chooses: on the drive home, during a daily walk, or during one's morning shower. Reflective exercises help one clarify one's thoughts and sift through what one has learned, and they indicate the need and ways to adjust behavior.

A school counselor leader and his/her mentor might add or substitute other strategies than those recommended here. The important point is to ensure some way of receiving ongoing feedback from oneself and others.

ANTICIPATED OUTCOMES

A solid understanding of the anticipated outcomes from the school counselor's successful improvement plan is imperative. "Begin with the end in mind." (Covey, 1989). This is Habit 2 from Covey's model of leadership described in *The 7 Habits of Highly Effective People*. In Covey's analogy of constructing a house, he states:

> You create it in every detail before you ever hammer the first nail into place. You try to get a very clear sense of what kind of house you want. If you want a family-centered home, you plan to put a family room where it would be a natural gathering place. You plan sliding glass doors and a patio for children to play outside. You work with your mind until you get a clear image of what you want to build (Covey, 1989, p. 99).

School counselor leaders must have a clear vision of what the improvement will look like. This gives them the incentive to continue with the learning and behavioral practices established for those times when things become difficult or they become lax in following through with their plan. It will be helpful to discuss this with their mentor during one of their early meetings. They can brainstorm all of the benefits that will accrue from achieving the objectives specified.

Self-Assessment and Exploration

In this exercise you will use the results of related exercises and self-assessments completed up to this point to develop a *leadership improvement plan* for one or more leadership behaviors.

Instructions: For each plan:

1. Identify a behavior or skill you wish to improve.
2. Review the results of relevant self-assessments you have completed earlier in this book. For example, if you want to improve your assertive behavior, review the results of your assertiveness self-assessment in Chapter 3.
3. List the objectives of your plan.
4. Designate an appropriate mentor (you may choose one mentor for all the plans or you may prefer to choose different mentors for different plans).
5. List your strategies for achieving your objectives.
6. List your strategies for monitoring your progress.
7. List from one to three anticipated outcomes. For example, if your objective is to be more assertive, one anticipated outcome might be that you will contribute a comment or suggestion in every leadership team meeting that you attend.

Leadership Improvement Plan 1 (behavior/skill to be improved)

_____

_____

Objectives:

1. _____

2. _____

3. _____

Mentor: _____

Strategies to achieve objectives:

1. _____

2. _____

3. _____

Strategies to monitor progress:

1. _____

2. _____

3. _____

Anticipated outcomes:

1. _____

2. _____

3. _____

Discuss the plan with a mentor and a learning partner. Incorporate useful ideas from your mentor and learning partner and schedule times with each of them to update them on your progress.

Leadership Improvement Plan 2 (behavior/skill to be improved)

_____

_____

Objectives:

1. _____

2. _____

3. _____

Mentor: _____

Strategies to achieve objectives:

1. _____

2. _____

3. _____

Strategies to monitor progress:

1. _____

2. _____

3. _____

Anticipated outcomes:

1. _____

2. _____

3. _____

Discuss the plan with a mentor and a learning partner. Incorporate useful ideas from your mentor and learning partner and schedule times with each of them to update them on your progress.

Leadership Improvement Plan 3 (behavior/skill to be improved)

_____

_____

Objectives:

1. _____

2. _____

3. _____

Mentor: _____

Strategies to achieve objectives:

1. _____

2. _____

3. _____

Strategies to monitor progress:

1. _____

2. _____

3. _____

Anticipated outcomes:

1. _____

2. _____

3. _____

Discuss the plan with a mentor and the colleague or learning partner who agreed to observe your leadership behavior. Incorporate useful ideas from your mentor and colleague or learning partner and schedule times with each of them to update them on your progress.

CHAPTER SUMMARY

This chapter focused on how to benefit from the results of self-assessments for leadership development. Self-assessments can be enjoyable but are useful to school counselors as educational leaders only if counselors analyze the results and identify areas that need improvement. The chapter also introduced a model for a leadership improvement plan. A good basic improvement plan includes objectives, strategies for achieving the objectives, and strategies for monitoring progress. The selection of a mentor experienced in leadership is important to the success of the plan. A mentor who successfully demonstrates the skill or behavior a counselor wants to improve is the best choice to guide and help the counselor to develop appropriate strategies for change.

One of Covey's 7 Habits of Highly Effective People is to "Begin with the end in mind" (Covey, 1989). Clearly articulating the expected change a counselor wants to see in himself or herself is a vital component of the school counselor's improvement plan. Knowing one's anticipated outcomes will serve to keep the school counselor leader on track while he/she strives to achieve identified goals and objectives.

Whether experienced as a leader or beginning to learn about leadership practices, one can benefit from continued self-discovery and practice. The leadership development plan is not designed to be a finished product but can be used continuously throughout a school counselor's career. As one discovers new things about oneself and new challenges present themselves, the school counselor can simply fill in the blanks and prepare for continued successes.

REVIEW AND REFLECT

1. Review the list of responsibilities of the counseling department chairperson presented in the counselor's story in this chapter. Make a list of all the leadership skills in which you currently feel competent that would contribute to your successful performance of such duties.

_____

_____

_____

_____

_____

_____

_____

2. Complete a daily leadership journal for one week. Set aside the time to journal observations of leadership behaviors in your daily activities and interactions. Describe your leadership behaviors and practices as you performed duties and interacted with others. Did you create or take advantage of opportunities to practice new leadership behaviors? At the end of the week, discuss your journal entries with a learning partner or colleague. Share what you learned about your developing leadership style.

Observations	_Comments_
Monday	
_____	_____
_____	_____
_____	_____
_____	_____
_____	_____

Observations	Comments
Tuesday	
Wednesday	
Thursday	
Friday	

RELEVANT WEBSITES

American School Counselor Association: www.schoolcounselor.org
American Counselor Association: www.aca.org
American Educational Research Association: www.aera.net

REFERENCES

Bolman, L. G., & Deal, T. E. (2001). *Leading with soul.* San Francisco, CA: Jossey-Bass.

Bolman, L. G., & Deal, T. E. (2002). *Reframing the path to school leadership.* Thousand Oaks, CA: Corwin Press, Inc.

Covey, S. R. (1989). *The 7 habits of highly effective people.* New York: Simon & Schuster.

DeVoss, J. A., & Andrews, M. F. (2003). A new model for leadership and advocacy training in counselor education. *Arizona Counseling Journal, 23,* 7–13.

Kouzes, J. M., & Posner, B. Z. (2001). *Leadership practices inventory facilitators guide.* San Diego, CA: Jossey-Bass/Pfeiffer.

Miles, M., & Miles, A. (1982). *The leadership manual.* Unpublished manuscript.

CHAPTER 8
Leadership Challenges Ahead

A QUEST TO PROMOTE THE SCHOOL COUNSELING VISION

Brian had been a school counselor for only three years when he realized the large amount of time he was spending in his school as an educational leader. He was greatly impressed with the need for leadership in the school counseling field, and not just leadership for a chosen few. Brian knew that if school counselors were serious about accomplishing the vision of the Transforming School Counseling Initiative (1999), leadership behavior had to become a way of life for all school counselors. It had to become integrated into their daily activities in schools. It was already happening and having an impact on him and his colleagues.

To promote his vision of school counselors as leaders and leadership by example, Brian decided to get involved at the state level on the governing board of his state school counselors' association. He helped develop a website for the organization, thereby increasing the organization's ability to communicate to a wider audience and to create a constant presence in the school counseling community. He was elected as president of the state school counselor organization. He organized the first state organization research summit to promote data collection and analysis to demonstrate the difference that school counseling makes to K–12 children.

In addition to his involvement in the state school counselors' organization, Brian committed himself to completing a doctoral program in educational leadership. He felt this degree would help to hone his already well-developed leadership skills and provide him with greater knowledge of research design and statistical analysis to help with the school counseling research he was doing and promoting with others.

Case Discussion

Questions About This Case

- What were some of the key issues that this school counselor addressed?
- What beliefs did Brian develop that guided him to accept leadership roles?
- Can a school counselor be effective without developing and applying leadership skills?
- What messages about school counselor roles and priorities does this scenario convey?
- What can we learn from this case example about working with other school personnel?

Further Thoughts on This Case

Brian's vision of school counseling became a source of inspiration to other practicing school counselors, counselor and educational leadership educators, district school guidance coordinators, and school administrators around the state as they increased the degree to which they collaborated on research studies and other projects. It was Brian's belief that the key to progress was making connections with other school counselors and K–12 stakeholders with similar visions and commitments to the missions of the school and the school counseling profession.

CHAPTER OBJECTIVES

School counselors face numerous leadership challenges: continuing to clarify role definition, obtaining optimal training, integrating programming, defining delivery systems, choosing a generalist versus specialist role, attaining reasonable student-to-counselor ratios, accepting leadership, taking on advocacy and public relations roles, developing technological competencies, and continuing involvement in professional development.

The objectives of this chapter are to:

1. Provide a perspective on the professional challenges ahead for school counselors with suggestions for addressing them.
2. Provide a perspective on the systemic challenges for school counselors with suggestions for initiating systemic change.

KEY PROFESSIONAL CHALLENGES: CURRENT AND FUTURE

The school counseling profession faces a challenge to define and enunciate its roles and functions more clearly as social changes and socioeconomic pressures influence the changing directions of school programs. The next generation of counselors has an opportunity to be significant contributors to the responses the schools make to these demands (Baker, 2000, p. v).

Professional school counseling's development over its history of more than a hundred years was influenced by a variety of forces, including the industrial revolution's exploitation of children, population immigration and migration, the educational reform movement at the turn of the 20th century, the evolution of counseling theory, and the national agenda. At the turn of the 21st century, educational reform once again has become a primary influence on the evolution of this profession.

Several authors have identified and discussed current and future challenges for school counseling (Baker, 2000; Gysbers, 2001; Paisley & Borders, 1995; Paisley & McMahon, 2001; Sandhu, 2001; Sears & Granello, 2002). In addition, a group of about 300 counselors, counselor educators, central office personnel, and state-level personnel who attended a national conference, Leading and Managing Comprehensive School Guidance Programs, in February 2002, in Greensboro, North Carolina, listed ten critical issues in school counseling (American School Counselor Association, 2002). These key professional and systemic challenges and issues facing school counselors are addressed in this chapter and organized by topics. Under the main heading of professional challenges are: school counselor role definition, school counselor preparation, generalist versus specialist roles, technological competencies, and professional development. Under the heading of systemic challenges are: school counseling programming, school counseling program delivery system, reasonable student-to-counselor ratios, and leadership/advocacy/public relations.

School Counselor Role Definition

Role definition has been frequently identified as a challenge for the school counseling profession and has caused considerable difficulty in daily practice and limited credibility for the profession. Perceptions of school counselor roles vary widely even within the same school district. Some school counselors have reported experiencing a lack of administrative support, confusing expectations, and lack of respect (ASCA, 2002). Sears and Granello (2002) noted that school counselors struggle with role definition. Paisley and Borders (1995) stated that school counselors experience lack of control over day-to-day activities and sometimes competing expectations from principals and counseling directors. In *School Counseling for the Twenty-first Century,* Baker (2000) stated, "School counseling, long viewed by some as an ancillary service in the schools, remains unclearly defined both within and outside the profession" (p. v). It is important for school counselor roles to be clear yet broad-ranged and not so demanding that they limit effectiveness.

In the early stages of the Transforming School Counseling Initiative, House and Martin, of the Education Trust (1998), outlined the new-vision school counselor role and compared it to the traditional role of school counselor (see Table 1-1 in Chapter 1). The new-vision school counselor is expected to be a proactive leader who is committed to high-quality education and equal access to higher education for all students. The school counselor is envisioned as an assertive advocate and social activist on behalf of students, parents, schools, and the school counseling profession.

In an effort to assist school counselors in defining their roles more clearly, ASCA adopted position statements regarding the profession. In one statement concerning uncredentialed school counseling personnel, ASCA (1990) emphasized that school counselors should be expected to lead in creating, organizing, and implementing school counseling program activities for both credentialed and uncredentialed personnel. Good graduate training programs prepare school counselors to lead their school's counseling program.

School Counselor Preparation

In order to carry out the mission of schools effectively and function optimally as part of school leadership teams, school counselor trainees must receive adequate training. Potential school counselors can choose from a variety of training programs. With information about the criteria for high-quality graduate training, they should be able to identify graduate programs that meet the national standards of the Council for the Accreditation of Counseling and Related Educational Programs (CACREP, 2001). State departments of education are adopting CACREP standards as minimum standards for certification or licensure (Baker, 2000; Sears & Granello, 2002).

Even with CACREP standards, there has been little consistency across school counseling training programs. In 1992, although 195 graduate programs in 72 institutions were accredited by CACREP (Kandor & Bobby, 1992), the programs varied considerably in curriculum from one program to another. CACREP standards (2001) for master's-level school counseling programs require a minimum of 48 semester hours of graduate study in the following eight areas: professional identity, social and cultural diversity, human growth and development, career development, helping relationships, group work, assessment, and research and program evaluation. In addition, CACREP specifies that school counselor trainees must successfully complete a 100-hour practicum and a 600-hour internship in school settings. *These are considered minimal standards for counselor preparation.*

ASCA (2000) developed a list of school counselor competencies which fall into three domains: knowledge competencies, skill competencies, and professional competencies.

Some examples of the knowledge competencies are human development theories and concepts, career decision-making theories and techniques, and program development models. Some of the skill competencies include: diagnosing student needs, career and educational counseling, and planning and conducting in-service training sessions for staff. Professional competencies include: conducting a self-evaluation to determine strengths and areas needing improvement, advocating for appropriate state and national legislation, and adopting a set of professional ethics to guide practice. It is in the best interest of prospective school counseling students to seek graduate programs that are CACREP-accredited, have been continuously updated and aligned with national standards and the Transforming School Counseling Initiative and that provide some formal leadership skills training.

In addition to the school counselor competencies, ASCA (2000) identified a list of personal attributes of successful school counselors. Some of the characteristics include: a genuine interest in the welfare of others, openness to learning, willingness to take risks, a strong sense of self-worth, caring and warmth, and a keen sense of humor. Some of these characteristics can be acquired during the course of training whereas others are innate. The complete list of effective school counselor skill competencies and personal characteristics is available from ASCA.

Self-Assessment and Exploration

The purpose of this exercise is to briefly assess yourself in two of the three ASCA competency areas: personal attributes and knowledge in school counseling.

1. Circle the degree to which you possess and demonstrate the personal attributes and competencies of successful school counselors listed below.
2. Based on your score (maximum = 30 for personal attributes, maximum = 40 for knowledge), note how closely you resemble the successful school counselor.
3. List areas for improvement on your leadership improvement plan.

Personal Attributes   (1 = very unlike you   5 = very like you)

Interest in welfare of others	1	2	3	4	5	
Openness to learning	1	2	3	4	5	
Willingness to take risks	1	2	3	4	5	
Strong sense of self-worth	1	2	3	4	5	
Caring and warmth	1	2	3	4	5	
Keen sense of humor	1	2	3	4	5	*Score* _____

Knowledge   (1= very little knowledge   5 = very knowledgable)

Human development theories and concepts	1	2	3	4	5	
Career decision-making theories and techniques	1	2	3	4	5	
Professional identity	1	2	3	4	5	
Social and cultural diversity	1	2	3	4	5	
Helping relationships	1	2	3	4	5	
Group dynamics	1	2	3	4	5	
Assessment principles	1	2	3	4	5	
Research and program evaluation	1	2	3	4	5	*Score* _____

How closely do you fit the ideal? Note areas to address in your leadership improvement plan.

_____

_____

_____

_____

Generalist Versus Specialist Roles

School counselors face the decision of whether they are generalists or specialists. It may be best to make this decision based on the needs of the school district or individual school and the decision may be influenced by the degree to which teams are utilized. If the school has a counseling department, the professional school counselors may be expected to be part of the departmental team. In the new-vision role (House & Martin, 1998), the school counselor is likely to be a member and/or leader of one or more school leadership teams (for example, staff development planning, suicide prevention, or crisis response).

Such teams can operate in a variety of ways. In some settings, the most efficient teamwork occurs when members are specialists who continuously hone specific knowledge bases and related skills. In the case of a counseling department team, the counselors might divide the departmental responsibilities depending on the special qualifications of its members. In other settings, professional school counselor team members work optimally as generalists and provide an array of services to preassigned caseloads of students. In some environments, a department may operate most efficiently with some specialists and some generalists.

When a school has only one counselor assigned, that counselor is most likely to function as a generalist. This is frequently the case for elementary school counselors. These school counselors can become isolated if they are not proactive in getting involved on leadership teams and in other collaborative relationships.

Technological Competence

Currently, competence in the use of technology for school counselors is clearly an expectation (Sandhu, 2001). The Association for Counselor Education and Supervision (ACES) Technology Interest Network (1999) established twelve technological competencies for counselors that should be included in counselor education. These competencies, which are expected to need updating continuously, are summarized here. Counselors need to be able to perform the tasks listed in the checklist in Box 8-1.

Sabella and Tyler (Sandhu, 2001) provide a detailed description and discussion of each of these competencies. School counselors who have stayed current in their profession recognize that up-to-date technology skills are necessary tools supporting effective school counseling work.

Self-Assessment of Technology Competence

Evaluate your technological competence using the checklist provided in Box 8-1. How many of the 12 school counselor technological competencies on the checklist provided have you mastered? If there are some in which you are lacking, how can you go about achieving at least basic competency? Write a plan to improve your technological competence and add it to your leadership improvement plan.

Professional Development

Due to the rapidly changing educational environment, professional development is a priority for counselors in schools. School counselors can utilize professional development opportunities to stay current in the profession and maintain their professional identity. Professional development is an opportunity to network and exchange

---

Box 8-1   Checklist of Technological Competencies for Counselors

_____ 1. Use productivity software to develop web pages, group presentations, letters, and reports.

_____ 2. Use audiovisual equipment such as video recorders, audio recorders, projection equipment, videoconferencing equipment, and playback units.

_____ 3. Use computerized statistical packages.

_____ 4. Use computerized testing, diagnostic, and career decision-making programs with clients.

_____ 5. Use e-mail.

_____ 6. Help clients search for various types of counseling-related information via the Internet, including information about careers, employment opportunities, educational and training opportunities, financial assistance/scholarships, treatment procedures, and social and personal information.

_____ 7. Subscribe, participate in, and sign off counseling-related listservs.

_____ 8. Use counseling-related CD-ROM databases.

_____ 9. Know strengths and weaknesses of counseling services provided via the Internet.

_____ 10. Know the legal and ethical codes that relate to counseling services via the Internet.

_____ 11. Use the Internet for finding and using continuing education opportunities in the school counseling profession.

_____ 12. Evaluate the quality of Internet information.

Technology Interest Network, 1999.

---

innovative ideas with other counseling professionals. State requirements for maintaining certification are another reason to continue one's professional development.

School counselors are encouraged to become members of at least one professional organization. Less than half of all school counselors take advantage of such membership. The benefits may include subscriptions to the publications of the organization, liability insurance discounts, notices of professional development opportunities, and networking opportunities as well as discounts on conferences and professional publications. These organizations offer potential leadership roles for school counselors along with the opportunity to make a difference at a systemic level. ASCA is the national professional school counselor organization and each state also has a state school counselor association.

SYSTEMIC CHALLENGES FOR SCHOOL COUNSELOR LEADERS

In addition to professional challenges, school counselors face a variety of systemic challenges in their schools, districts, and greater communities. The following sections address some of the major current and future systemic challenges for school counselors including: school counseling programming, the program delivery system, reasonable student-to-counselor ratios, and leadership/advocacy/public relations efforts.

Characteristics of Effective School Counseling Programs

Hart and Jacobi (1992) identified six problems with school counseling programs. In a presentation at the Education Trust Summer Academy, in Chicago in 2002, Mark Kuranz, a past president of ASCA, reminded participants of those six problems:

1. Lack of basic philosophy
2. Poor integration
3. Insufficient student access
4. Inadequate services for some students
5. Lack of counselor accountability
6. Failure to utilize other resources

Basic Philosophy

Kuranz noted, with a sense of urgency for the continued existence of the profession, that school counselors need to clearly tie their efforts to academic achievement. If school counseling programs in K–12 settings are going to survive, it is imperative that they be systematically planned and focused on the desired academic results rather than the traditional basis of services offered. The basic philosophy and mission of a school counseling program should follow directly from the school's mission. Examples of desired results might include improved national and state test results, improved graduation rates, improved attendance, decreased dropout rates, increased enrollment in postsecondary education programs, and increased enrollment of poor and minority students in high-level math and advanced placement (AP) courses.

Integrated, Longitudinal Developmental Counseling

Integration is a key characteristic of an effective school counseling program. An effectively integrated program needs to be longitudinal (Herr & Cramer, 1996) and should span from elementary school through secondary school. Furthermore, Sandhu (2001) stressed a holistic perspective, in which counseling programs, starting with elementary school, need to emphasize the interconnections among the cognitive, physical, and social development of children. In their book *Developing and Managing Your School Guidance Program,* Gysbers and Henderson (2000) described in detail the steps in designing a comprehensive guidance program for a school or district. The process involves concretely describing the content, organizational framework, time allotted, and resources needed. It is a time-intensive process but well worth the investment for the program. Studer (2005) provides a program development checklist.

For maximum effectiveness and relevance to all students, Sandhu (2001) recommends that school counseling programs be proactive and positive in approach. It is reasonable to design these programs to be comprehensive and well integrated into the mission of the school. Gysbers and Henderson (2000) reported that comprehensive guidance programs are becoming a reality in school districts across the United States. These programs are staffed by professional school counselors concerned with serving all students rather than focusing only on high- and low-achieving students and providing no or less-than-adequate services to all others.

Student Accessibility/Services for All Students

The national standards developed by the ASCA for school counseling programs are the essential elements of an effective school counseling program at any level of K–12 education. They address program content and expected knowledge, attitudes, and skill competencies for all students in schools with comprehensive school counseling programs. Three content areas include academic, career, and personal/social development. Under each of these headings are three standards which describe the outcomes for students of an effective school counseling program. For example, in the career development domain, standard B states, "Students will employ strategies to achieve future career success and satisfaction." The trifold developmental focus, including career development, should start in the elementary school and continue through twelfth grade (Sandhu, 2001).

Gysbers and Henderson (2000) described in detail how to adapt a school counseling program model to meet the specific needs of a school or a school district and to balance the use of the professional school counselor's time according to predetermined priorities. The use of established steering and school-community advisory committees is recommended throughout the decision-making process. This collaborative approach ensures that the school counseling program adopted by the decision makers will adequately address the systemic needs of the district or school.

The ASCA National Model (2003) for school counseling programs, as described in detail in Chapter 2, includes four major components: program foundation, delivery system, management system, and accountability. The model has a threefold emphasis on advocacy, leadership, and systemic change in keeping with themes of the school counseling reform movement. It provides school counselors with a framework for the development of school counseling programs while allowing flexibility for responsiveness to local community needs.

School counseling programs are responsible for guidance of all students. This means that counselors in the 21st century must be prepared to provide appropriate school counseling services to students and families of diverse cultural and ethnic backgrounds, those with learning disabilities, those with various sexual orientations, those with emotional and physical disabilities, and those with diverse religious beliefs and practices (Sandhu, 2001). It also means that school counselors need to meet the challenge to become assertive advocates for all students, especially disadvantaged and minority students, in the important work of closing the achievement gap between disadvantaged and minority students and their peers.

Gysbers (2001) contends that school counselors can reach all students through comprehensive school counseling programs with planned guidance activities in the classrooms. He cited research indicating that comprehensive guidance programs benefit students academically, in career development, and in school climate.

Currently, stage models of development are the foundation for school counseling programs. However, some leaders in the school counseling field question the adequacy of these models for this purpose (Green & Keys, 2001; Sears & Granello, 2002). The models may not sufficiently take into account issues of diversity and other contextual factors that are important when developing a school counseling program.

To address these concerns, Green and Keys (2001) recommend use of a development-in-context paradigm in school counseling program design. This model takes into consideration contextual factors such as culture, values, and living environment, that affect student development. School counselors operating from this model facilitate student awareness of self-in-context, an awareness of the multiple contexts affecting the student's life.

Although the profession emphasizes the role of school counselors in the delivery of comprehensive guidance programs, it has been noted that there are many obstacles (Sandhu, 2001). Although the comprehensive guidance approach is preplanned, proactive, and comprehensive in nature, in practice the school counselor must constantly strive to achieve and maintain balance in the school counseling program. Despite the best planning efforts, there continue to be many demands on the school counselor's time and effort. Sears and Granello (2002) noted that school counselors are pulled in different directions as they attempt to conform to national agenda. School counselors continue to respond to school-based crises and intervene on behalf of intensely disturbed, emotionally troubled students. Baker (2001) acknowledged many demands to which counselors in schools are expected to respond. Fortunately, the National Model and standards as well as the national, state, and local school counseling organizations are resources available to help school counselors meet the challenges of setting and assertively maintaining priorities for their school counseling programs.

Accountability

Baker (2000) explained the difference between the terms *evaluation* and *accountability*. "Evaluation is the act of gathering information about one's services; accountability is the act of reporting the results of the evaluation." He described basic school counselor accountability competencies, such as how to do a needs assessment and how to assess cost-effectiveness.

Accountability is expected of all educators, including school counselors. Data from their schools are easily available for school counselors to use in evaluating the impact of school counseling programs. School counselors have made progress and will continue to be expected to access and disaggregate data for developing data-driven school counseling programs. When school counselors report the outcomes of their interventions on achievement data, other educators begin to understand the connection between counseling programs and the mission of schools. In 1970, in the midst of economically difficult times, Arbuckle (1970/2000) wrote an article entitled "Does the School Really Need Counselors?" The article challenged the profession to become more accountable. In response, some individuals developed models for accountability; others reiterated the need for accountability; and some state legislation mandated accountability of school counseling. Yet many school counselors resisted instituting evaluation measures. Meanwhile, the pressure for school counseling program accountability mounted.

In the face of current educational reform and No Child Left Behind legislation that mandates educational accountability, school counselors can no longer afford to resist. With the economic stresses and decreased educational funding following the events of September 11, 2001, some school districts are asking Arbuckle's question. School counselors are challenged to advocate for their survival. Advocacy via use of data indicating the impact of school counseling programs on achievement can be powerful and gives the profession credibility.

The Need for Collaboration

Considering the challenge for school counselors to meet the needs of all children, the easiest way to serve students successfully may be through a team effort. Because typical school student-to-counselor ratios far exceed the ideal (between 200 and 300 to 1) (Baker, 2000), school counselors cannot adequately meet all students' needs without help. A recent ASCA study (2002) reported that in 1999–2000, the national average student-to-counselor ratio was 490 to 1. This lends support to the strategy of school counselors collaborating with others in the delivery of some guidance services to students.

Paisley and McMahon (2001) believe that school counselors must foster collaborative relationships with other school personnel, parents, professionals, and other community members in order to adequately meet student needs. By collaborating, school counselors enlarge the pool of talent and resources available to the school community. In some schools, teachers assist in effectively delivering the guidance curriculum in the classroom. It must be noted here that although the involvement of others in the counseling program can be beneficial to students, ethical and professional practice requirements (ASCA, 1998) dictate that counseling-related activities performed by uncredentialed personnel be supervised and coordinated by credentialed school counselors.

Self-Assessment and Exploration

In this exercise, you will identify the top three problems in your district or school and work on a plan for finding solutions.

Instructions: At the beginning of this section on school counseling programming, there is a list of six problems with school counseling programs identified by Mark Kuranz (2002).

A. Review the list and choose the top three problems in a school district with which you are familiar. If there are problems in your school or district that are not listed, put those on your top-three list.

Top Three Problems

1. _____

2. _____

3. _____

B. In small groups, share your lists. Then brainstorm possibilities for obtaining data about the problems and for approaching the problems.

Possible Sources of Data

1. _____

2. _____

3. _____

C. Identify key people to include on teams or committees involved in the problem-solving process.

Key People

1. _____

2. _____

3. _____

D. Make notes to take to school or district problem-solving meetings.

_____

_____

_____

_____

_____

School Counseling Program Delivery System

The *ASCA National Model* (2003) outlines the delivery system for school counseling programs. Based on this current national model, professional school counselors must be competent in the following areas in order to meet basic practice standards of the profession:

- Implementing developmental guidance curriculum
- Providing individual planning
- Offering responsive services to meet immediate needs
- Performing systems support administration and management activities

Currently, there is considerable consensus in the field of school counseling that the resources of the school counselor can be utilized best with a proactive developmental approach (Sandhu, 2001). The professional school counselor is expected to coordinate the design, planning, and implementation of the school counseling program with care and flexibility to adequately meet the needs of students, parents, teachers, administrators, and other stakeholders.

Reasonable Student-to-Counselor Ratios

Reasonable student-to-counselor ratios are a prerequisite for school counselors to become adequately familiar with students and their needs. Because of the amount of variation in type and intensity of need in student populations and in expectations of school counselors, it is difficult and unrealistic to determine a standard ratio of students-to-counselor to fit all settings.

However, generally, caseloads of 300 or fewer are seen as optimal (Baker, 2000). Student-to-counselor ratios are determined primarily by financial conditions and secondarily by the perceived value of the school counseling program (Shaw, 1973). Gysbers and Henderson (2000) offered a formula that calculates approximate student-to-counselor ratios in an optimal school counseling program. The ratio varies depending on the prearranged counseling program activities for the school and, therefore, the school counselor's availability to provide the program activities.

Leadership/Advocacy/Public Relations

Professional school counselors must successfully articulate to policy makers, media, and the public the essential contributions of school counselors to the mission of schools. In order to effectively educate the community about the important role of school counseling, professional school counselors must actively promote the profession and its mission. Baker (2000) suggests that social activism is the approach needed to achieve recognition of the preferred identity for professional school counselors. The Education Trust (1999) outlined the role of the new-vision school counselor as leader, advocate, collaborator, and consultant.

> The profession fosters conditions that ensure educational equity, access, and academic success for all students, K–12 . . . the trained school counselor must be an assertive advocate creating opportunities for all students. . . . The school counselor serves as a leader as well as an effective team member working with teachers, administrators, and other school personnel to make sure that each student succeeds. The school counselor as consultant empowers families to act on behalf of their children . . . as well as access available resources.

With a clearer definition of school counseling and the roles of professional school counselors, the local and national community can have a better understanding of the key contributions school counselors make in achieving educational equity for all children. Baker (2000) stressed that professional school counselors and their supporters need to join local and national professional organizations like ASCA, the Association for Counselor Education and Supervision (ACES), and the American Counseling Association (ACA) and initiate grassroots efforts to achieve dramatic educational change on a national level. He expressed concern that less than half of all school counselors are members of any professional organization.

CHAPTER SUMMARY

Professional school counseling in the United States has been influenced by a myriad of things, including: social reform efforts, immigration, economic changes, national defense issues, and the advancement of psychological and developmental theory. The impact of its evolution left the profession with numerous challenges at the end of the 20th century, including: clarifying the school counselor role definition, identifying and obtaining optimal school counselor preparation, deciding on generalist versus specialist roles, developing technological competencies, and participating in relevant professional development.

Furthermore, school counselors must address systemic challenges: integrating school counseling programming; clearly defining school counseling program delivery systems; attaining reasonable student-to-counselor ratios; and accepting leadership, advocacy, and public relations roles.

The role of the school counselor in the 21st century remains fluid and continually changing in response to the changing demands of our schools and our local and national communities. However, as the profession has continued the transformation process, it has sought to become actively involved in the educational reform movement, as opposed to its limited or nonexistent role in past reform movements. Counselors have begun to address the challenges and issues discussed in this chapter and are encouraged to continue this important work. In the process, school counselors have begun to speak as advocates with one voice to ensure that all students have equal access to a good education and, that in reality, no child is left behind.

REVIEW AND REFLECT

1. What school counseling organizations are you familiar with? do you belong to? Visit the websites of school counseling or related organizations and identify the benefits of belonging to such organizations. With a partner or small group, share the benefits of professional organization memberships that you have experienced personally or identified on websites such as www.schoolcounselor.org, www.aera.net, or www.aca.org. If you were not a member of at least one of these organizations prior to completing this exercise, are you planning to become a member? Share your rationale. Incorporate where appropriate in your leadership improvement plan.

2. Review one or more copies of *Professional School Counseling* and/or *Counseling Today* to identify at least two challenges faced by school counselors. Choose one of the challenges in which you can invest some time and effort and identify some actions you can take to help the profession address the challenge. For example, you can write a letter to an editor, become a member of a task force, or initiate a pilot project with a data-collection component.

   Share your ideas with a partner or small group and ask for feedback. Incorporate where appropriate in your leadership improvement plan.

RELEVANT WEBSITES

American School Counselor Association: www.schoolcounselor.org
American Counselor Association: www.aca.org
American Educational Research Association: www.aera.net

REFERENCES

American School Counselor Association. (1990). Role statement: The school counselor. *ASCA guide to membership resources*. Alexandria, VA: Author.

American School Counselor Association. (1998). *Ethical standards for school counselors*. Alexandria, VA: Author.

American School Counselor Association. (2000). *School counselor competencies* [Brochure]. Alexandria, VA: Author.

American School Counselor Association. (2002). ASCA study examines counselor-to-student ratios. *ASCA School Counselor, 39*(5), 50.

American School Counselor Association (2002). Hot topics for school counselors. *ASCA School Counselor, 39*(5), 51.

American School Counselor Association. (2003). *The ASCA national model: A framework for school counseling programs*. Alexandria, VA: Author.

Arbuckle, D. (2000). Does the school really need school counselors? In S. Baker (Ed.), *School counseling for the twenty-first century*. Upper Saddle River: NJ: Prentice Hall. (Original work published 1970)

Association for Counselor Education and Supervision (ACES) Technology Interest Network. (1999, April). *Technical competencies for counselor education students: Recommended guidelines for program development* [Online]. Available: www.chre.vt.edu/thohen/competencies.htm

Baker, S. (2000). *School counseling for the twenty-first century*. Upper Saddle River, NJ: Prentice Hall.

Campbell, C. A., & Dahir, C. A. (1997). *The national standards for school counseling programs*. Alexandria, VA: American School Counselor Association.

Council for the Accreditation of Counseling and Related Educational Programs (CACREP). (2001). *CACREP accreditation standards and procedures manual*. Alexandria, VA: Author.

Education Trust. (1999). *Transforming school counseling initiative* [Brochure]. Washington, DC: Author.

Green, A., & Keys, S. (2001). Expanding the developmental school counseling paradigm: Meeting the needs of the 21st century student. *Professional School Counseling, 5*, 84–95.

Gysbers, N. C. (2001). School guidance and counseling in the 21st century: Remember the past into the future. *Professional School Counseling, 5*, 96–105.

Gysbers, N. C., & Henderson, P. (2000). *Developing and managing your school guidance program*. Alexandria, VA: American Counseling Association.

Hart, P. J., & Jacobi, M. (1992). *From gatekeeper to advocate: Transforming the role of the school counselor*. New York: College Entrance Examination Board.

Herr, E. L., & Cramer, S. H. (1996). *Career guidance and counseling through the lifespan* (5th ed.). New York: HarperCollins.

House, R. M., & Martin, P. J. (1998). Advocating for better futures for all students: A new vision for school counselors. *Education, 119*, 284–291.

Kandor, J. R., & Bobby, C. L. (2000). Introduction to a special feature. In Baker, S. (Ed.). *School counseling for the twenty-first century*. Upper Saddle River: NJ: Prentice Hall. (Original work published 1992)

Kuranz, M. (2002, June). *The new ASCA national model for school counseling programs*. Presentation at the Education Trust 2002 Summer Academy, Chicago, IL.

Paisley, P. O., & Borders, L. D. (1995). School counseling: An evolving specialty. *Journal of Counseling and Development, 74*, 150–153.

Paisley, P. O., & McMahon, G. H. (2001). School counseling for the 21st century: Challenges and opportunities. *Professional School Counseling, 5*, 106–115.

Sandhu, D. H. (Ed.). (2001). *Elementary school counseling in the new millennium*. Alexandria, VA: American Counseling Association.

Sears, S. J., & Granello, D. H. (2002). School counseling now and in the future: A reaction. *Professional School Counseling, 5*, 164–171.

Shaw, M. C. (2000). School guidance systems: Objectives, functions, evaluation, and change. In S. Baker (Ed.), *School counseling for the twenty-first century*. Upper Saddle River NJ: Prentice Hall. (Original work published 1973)

Studer, J. R. (2005). *The professional school counselor*. Belmont, CA: Brooks/Cole.

CHAPTER 9
The School Counselor Advocate

A FAMILY LED TO COMMUNITY CONNECTIONS

William, an elementary school counselor in his second year of practice, had received a desperate phone call from a woman named Margaret, whose three grandchildren had recently come to live with her. The children were newly enrolled in his school. He asked her to come in during the lunch period the next day to talk about the children's needs. In their meeting, Margaret told William the story of how the children had come to live with her. She loved being a grandmother and greatly enjoyed her grandchildren. They were an important part of her life. Before they came to live with her, she had regular visits with them on Sunday afternoons and enjoyed the children's occasional overnight visits when her daughter and son-in-law needed a break. Margaret found grandparenting even more satisfying than parenting. Like many grandparents, she focused more on having fun with the children than training and disciplining them.

When her daughter, Dianna, called her one day to inform her that she and her husband, Robert, were divorcing, Margaret was shocked. Dianna explained that she and her husband had been having marital problems for more than a year. Dianna had kept the problems a secret from Margaret. Robert, a physician, had a serious substance abuse problem which required him to enter residential treatment for forty-five to sixty days. In addition to, and because of, Robert's substance abuse they also had serious financial problems.

Dianna had been struggling to hold the marriage and family together with little outside support. The stress had become overwhelming, and she had finally decided to file for divorce. She was extremely depressed and barely able to function and had even contemplated suicide.

The children exhibited both academic and behavioral problems. While with their parents, they attended school in the highly affluent geographical area of the city where the family resided. Dianna was too embarrassed to inform school personnel about her husband's substance abuse and their marital troubles. She finally built up the courage to tell her mother about all the problems and to ask her to take the children to live with her while she sought her own treatment for depression and located a job to support herself and eventually the children. If Robert were ever allowed to practice medicine again, it would be at least several years before he could pay off the debt he had acquired.

Margaret was unable to say no to her daughter's request. Despite her small home and limited income from Social Security, she took the three children in to live with her for approximately six months while her daughter received treatment and sought employment. She promptly enrolled the children in the elementary school in her lower-middle-class neighborhood. She met the principal, the school nurse, and the school counselor and informed them of the family problems that had led to her taking guardianship of the children. Her tone of voice relayed her sense of desperation. She hoped that the school counselor could facilitate the children's adjustment to their parents' divorce, to moving away from their parents and friends into a different neighborhood, to attending a new school, and to living in Margaret's crowded home with their newly-defined relationship with her and the newly-developed limits she had in place for them. She also hoped that, despite their adjustment issues, the children's academic performance in their new school would reflect their true potential.

Case Discussion

Questions About This Case

- What were some of the key issues that this school counselor needed to consider?
- What other resources could be tapped for the family described and others in similar circumstances?
- How can a school counselor identify targets for systemic change from daily contacts with students and their families?
- What messages about school counselor roles and priorities does this scenario convey?
- What can we learn from this case example about working with other resources in a school and the greater community?

Further Thoughts on This Case

The children and the family in the above example were clearly at risk and in need of a variety of services. Margaret was overwhelmed in her new role as parent of her grandchildren. As many parents and grandparents in her situation do, she sought help from the school, especially the school counselor. The school counselor on his/her own is not likely to be able to adequately meet such a family's multiple needs. However, there is much the counselor can do to influence the school environment to be responsive to the needs of the children and the family and other families like this one.

The school counselor can serve as an advocate and change agent on behalf of all children in the school by identifying and connecting such families with resources and helping to develop programs where there are no resources. For example, there is a need for support groups for the many grandparents currently in the position of raising grandchildren. The school counselor could be instrumental in helping to refer people to an existing group or to initiate such a group. In addition, the children could be invited to participate in groups for children of divorced parents. The children could be offered tutoring to help with their academics. Depending on the intensity of their behavioral problems, it might be appropriate for the school counselor to refer the children and family for outpatient therapy in a community mental health facility. The grandmother might qualify for food stamps and other social services to which the school counselor could direct her. The children might be paired with "buddies" in the school, other students in their grades who could show them around, introduce them to people, and generally make them feel more welcome in the new school setting.

CHAPTER OBJECTIVES

The objectives for this chapter are to:

1. Define and discuss the concept of advocacy relative to the role of the school counselor as educational leader.
2. Address the need for advocacy for students, school personnel, schools, districts, educational causes, and the profession of school counseling.
3. Present a model for school counselor advocacy that incorporates principles of effective educational leadership.

WHAT IS ADVOCACY AND WHO CAN BE AN ADVOCATE?

In their textbook, *The School Counselor in the Twenty-first Century*, Baker and Gerler (2004) discuss the school counselor as an advocate. "Like it or not, the schools have become more than a place to impart knowledge. They have become, seemingly more than before, one institution that must help victims or potential victims of debilitating social problems, using both reactive and proactive responses. School counselors have a place in this scene as collaborators with other professional colleagues. School counseling was born in the social reform movement of another era, the legacy lives on, and it will continue to flourish" (p. 289).

According to the Education Trust (1999), "Advocacy is the process of reducing the effect of environmental and institutional barriers that impede student success." This statement is an essential part of the Education Trust's (2002) redefinition of the school counseling profession. Homan (1999) described advocacy as a change-producing process that affects attitudes, policies, or practices in order to reduce problems or improve the meeting of student needs.

Advocacy efforts of school counselors focus on promoting equity for students. In this context equity means providing what students need to be successful. The needs of one student can vary greatly from those of another student. Some students require considerably more than others in order to achieve academic success. Therefore, it is important to note that equity does not mean providing the same resources for everyone.

According to the *American Heritage Dictionary* (2001), an advocate is "one that argues for a cause," "one that pleads in another's behalf." Lee and Walz (1998) defined an advocate in a school context as someone who intervenes in students' lives and in the world. Eldridge (1983) described an advocate as one who takes action on issues that have an impact on students. The Education Trust (2000) noted three common forms of advocacy in counseling: advocacy for clients, advocacy for systems change, and advocacy for the counseling profession. Lee and Walz (1998) emphasized the mandate for counselors to be involved in social action. They stated that social action is based on two premises. First, the environment plays a critical role in determining behavior. And, second, counselors are socially, morally, and professionally responsible for addressing social issues.

When school counselors serve as leaders and advocates, they can empower themselves, students, parents, school personnel, and others to "collaborate in the service of shared visions, values and missions" (Bolman & Deal, 1994) to accomplish change at any level. Every student, regardless of race, culture, ethnicity, religious orientation, or socioeconomic status, is entitled to access to success. School counselors can utilize their unique skills and training toward eliminating environmental obstacles to social justice. To be effective in their professional mission, school counselors not only can but must play an active part in addressing societal issues.

Menacker (1976) noted that counselors can identify harmful institutional policies and actively seek to change them. Counselors who accept the roles of activist and advocate take risks on behalf of their clients. To be effective while taking such risks, school counselors need to use their skills in diplomacy to minimize negative responses from teachers and administrators (Ponzo, 1974). Counselor advocates must be skilled in identifying allies and enlisting support from others. They must be assertive leaders.

Baker and Gerler (2004) included a chapter on advocacy in their text on school counseling. They noted that the environment is sometimes the source of a student's problems, and when this is the case traditional counseling efforts are ineffective. Instead, counselors need to advocate for client assistance, influencing the environment to better meet the client's needs.

Further support for school counselors as advocates is provided in the standards of the Council on Accreditation for Counseling and Related Educational Programs (CACREP, 2001). These standards state that school counselors need to be knowledgeable about opportunities that enhance student success and the barriers that impede student success.

Students' needs may be as basic as food, appropriate clothing, school supplies, and transportation. Other needs stem from systemic barriers within the educational environment and may not be as obvious. For example, minority students may not be encouraged to take advanced placement and other challenging classes and may not be adequately prepared for college. If educational leaders maintain that all students should have the option of a college education, the inadequate preparation of some groups of students is an injustice. Regardless of the type of need, it is necessary for the school counselor to be an active responder and advocate for students. In addition to circumstantial and educational environment barriers to student success, students (and all members of society) face continuously mounting stress from war, terrorism, and other frightening world, national, and local events. Not surprisingly, school counselors have experienced increased demands to act as student advocates.

ADVOCATING FOR LEGISLATIVE ACTION

Instructions: Go online to the ASCA home page at www.schoolcounselor.org. Locate the Legislative Updates page and review it. Summarize two important pieces of proposed legislation and share your critique of their pros and cons with your learning group. Describe where the legislation is in the process of being reviewed so that learning group members can contact their members of Congress and/or senators to share their views.

Characteristics and Skills of an Effective Advocate

Ponzo (1974) recommended that counselor advocates be flexible and willing to compromise; understanding of themselves and others and willing to learn from the system; and skilled at setting realistic goals. Effective advocates develop leadership and advocacy capabilities from within, by building on their strengths, and identify targets for change by paying attention to the external environment. A useful guide to advocacy for the new school counselor is the advocacy model developed and recently revised by the Education Trust (2002, 2003). The Education Trust's National Center for Transforming School Counseling (NCTSC) in Washington, D.C., has prepared a cadre of trainers from various regions of the United States to deliver NCTSC professional development to school district personnel throughout the country. (Information about the five-module training that is delivered in four days over several months can be obtained by contacting the Educational Trust at the web address provided at the end of this chapter.) This advocacy approach is delineated in seven preliminary steps and six action steps for systems change (Box 9-1).

Seven Preliminary Steps for Systemic Change

The seven preliminary steps for change were designed to help counselors in a school or district to identify issues warranting systemic change. This type of change requires looking at school issues beyond individual case scenarios. However, the advocacy process may start as a result of one or more disturbing case scenarios that stir school counselors and other staff to look at the big picture or systems aspects of those individual cases. The case presented at the beginning of this chapter is an example of a situation that may warrant a closer examination of potential systemic issues in a school or district.

Box 9-1 Advocacy in Thirteen Steps

Preliminary Steps	1. Identify the problem and the extent of the problem using data. 2. Determine systemic contributions to the problem. 3. Assess the risks of action versus inaction. 4. Identify allies. 5. Identify opportunities to address the problem through teaming and collaboration. 6. Work with allies to clarify the source and focus of the problem. 7. Gather additional data to support the need for change.
Action Steps	8. Delineate an action plan and take only realistic action. 9. Identify policies/practices that need to change and develop change strategies. 10. Enlist the support of influential people and policy makers. 11. Identify sources of resistance and develop strategies for addressing/challenging it. 12. Evaluate progress and revise the plan as needed. 13. Share the results.

Adapted from the Education Trust, 2003.

Step 1: Identify the Problem and the Extent of the Problem Using Data

How do you identify a problem to be targeted for change? There are numerous issues of concern in any school. In some schools and districts, it may be a challenge to choose from the numerous problems that need to be addressed. As you consider a target for change, it is necessary to review district and school data that indicate the extent of the problem.

In the search for a target for systemic change, you can use informal and formal approaches as you begin to gather information about school problems that create barriers to student achievement. It is worthwhile to gain several perspectives on school issues and then to compare verbalized concerns with corresponding data. A few hours spent in the teachers' lounge listening to themes of concern can be of value. Board of education meetings may be a useful source of board and parent concerns. A needs assessment in which students, parents, faculty, and staff complete anonymous questionnaires regarding problems and potential solutions can provide valuable insights. You and the other stakeholders of your school and district are likely to have additional insights and approaches for identifying a target for change.

Before making a commitment to target a specific problem for change, it is important to examine existing data to determine the extent of the problem. The school district's data system can be of assistance. Schools and individuals within specific schools may also have data that shed light on the problem. In addition to determining the extent of the problem, take time to assess the problem's importance and how much of an impact a solution will have on the educational system.

In order to determine how widespread a problem may be, you can look at existing data to verify the existence and impact of the problem. Does the issue currently affect a few or a large number of students? Has it affected only a few students at any one time but a large number of students when the issue is examined over the course of time? The issue may seem at first glance to have a negligible impact, but on closer examination it may be a major problem for a school or district. How often is it brought up by stakeholders? How many people have recognized it as an issue? Is it limited in its effects or does it affect more that one area of the school's functioning? Is it a new problem brought on by change in the school or district or an old problem continuing to rear its head?

If existing data does not answer your questions about how widespread the problem is, you may need to gather some additional data. You can collect both quantitative and qualitative data to provide a thorough understanding of the issue. Seek out others who are interested in helping to collect data or who, without your prior knowledge, have already collected data on the problem.

Step 2: Determine Systemic Contributions to the Problem

In order to address this issue, you will need to review district and school policies and become familiar with the practices and attitudes. Consider whether the problem may have been created by school or district policies, practices, or attitudes. Question as to whether it is maintained or worsened by these policies, practices, or attitudes. And, in any case, consider what specific policies, practices, or attitudes need to change to address the problem.

Step 3: Assess the Risks of Action Versus Inaction

It is important to explore some of the potential consequences of taking action on the issue. What is likely to happen if no action is taken? Who will be affected by action? Who will be affected by inaction? Are there risks of action versus no action? What are some perceived benefits that might result from addressing the problem? What will it cost in terms of time, energy, and money? What other costs are there in pursuing change on this particular issue? Weigh the costs versus the potential benefits of change.

Step 4: Identify Allies

As you seek to identify allies, you will want to ask, Who, if anyone, is already working on the problem? Who needs to be involved? Who are the stakeholders who have power and influence to see the process through the stages of change? Is there already a task force or committee that exists to address such issues? Who has an interest and time and energy to contribute to addressing the problem?

Step 5: Identify Opportunities for Teaming and Collaboration

Teaming occurs when a group of educational professionals with a common task come together to accomplish that task. The focus is on the task. Examples of teaming in schools include: high school counseling department meetings, dropout prevention committees, and science department meetings. Teaming is frequently mandated by virtue of one's role in a school or district, for example, high school counselor, dropout prevention specialist, or science teacher.

Collaboration occurs when a group of people work together toward a common goal. The focus is on relationships that enrich the process of goal achievement.

Collaboration frequently involves pooling the resources of a diverse group of stake-holders that mirrors the characteristics of the school and local community. Collaboration generally occurs when a person or group of people seek out other people with the same goal who possess qualities that will enhance the group's efforts. Collaboration is generally actively initiated and a voluntary process.

When seeking opportunities for teaming and collaboration, consider already existing teams and collaborative groups that may be focused on related tasks and goals. In addition, seek potential collaborators who possess knowledge or abilities needed by the group. The Education Trust (2003) recommends seeking potential collaborators who have one or more of the following qualities: social and/or political credibility/influence, natural leadership abilities, technical competence, authority, the ability to allocate resources, and diverse perspectives.

Step 6: Clarify the Source and Focus of the Problem

It is useful for a collaborative group focused on systems change to have a discussion with a larger group of stakeholders who are concerned about the issue. Start with a review of all relevant data on hand. The collaborative group for systems change can facilitate discussion in the larger group. To the best of the group's ability and given the data available, the focus of the discussion should be determining the source of systemic contributions to the target problem.

The collaborators-for-change group can follow a systematic process designed to achieve a consensus regarding the focus for systemic change. As the collaborators-for-change group facilitates the discussion of stakeholders, the group can actively promote consensus building through a process of group decision making in which the active consent of all group members is required before closure is reached. Consensus does not equal majority rule, where only one more than half of the members must consent to reach a decision. With a large group of stakeholders, it is useful to divide into small groups to brainstorm the sources of systemic contributions to the problem and ask each small group to report the group's top three sources with the rationale for each choice. As each group reports, a facilitator should record the responses for each group on a flip chart, whiteboard, or chalkboard.

After making the list of systemic contributions, narrow it down within the context of group discussion. Find items on the list that all members agree can be combined and other items that can be eliminated from the list based on low priority. Once you have narrowed down the list, ask each person to rank order their top three items from the remaining list and note the individual rankings next to each item. Often, at this point in the process, there will be a few items that have a lot of support and other items that have little or no support. Continue to facilitate the discussion, combining and eliminating items with all group members' consent until the entire group agrees on a focus for systemic change.

The following rules guide the process of consensus building:

- There is no voting or quantitative method used to reach consensus.
- Any one person can veto the rank ordering if that person strongly opposes it.
- The group should work toward integrating everyone's ideas and opinions.

Step 7: Gather Additional Data to Support the Need for Change

The collaborative group that is working for systems change will need to determine whether the existing data are sufficient or if there is a need for additional data. If further data are necessary, the group needs to determine exactly what data are important, how to collect the data, and who will collect it. The collaborative group should determine what type of data it will need to support the proposed change addressing the targeted issue. Furthermore, the group will need to determine the type of data needed by decision makers, funding sources, and the collaborative group itself.

Six Action Steps for Systemic Change

When a problem has been identified and found to warrant action for systemic change, the following six action steps can be taken to assure a thorough and systematic approach. The use of such an approach is likely to increase the odds of success in the work of advocacy that is often met with great resistance. It is the tendency of systems to maintain the status quo and to resist efforts to disrupt that state. The six action steps in advocating for systemic change are described in the following sections. The numbering of the steps will continue from the seven preliminary steps, starting with Step 8.

Step 8. Delineate an Action Plan and Take Only Realistic Action

With the stakeholders/allies, the collaborative group working for systems change will need to develop a detailed action plan. List all action steps that need to be taken to initiate, implement, and maintain the desired change. The group may want to begin the process by brainstorming all possible action steps without evaluating them. Once a complete list is developed, the collaborative group can review and critique each proposed step. The group may determine that some steps are unrealistic and may decide to eliminate them from the list. It may decide to combine some proposed steps that are similar. The steps that remain after the evaluation process can be prioritized based on criteria including: the amount of impact they have on the issue, the ease with which they can be implemented, and the cost and availability of resources and money.

The collaborative group must consider a variety of factors such as school/district and state priorities, responses to the proposed change agenda from supporters and detractors, and resources available to determine which actions steps are realistic and which rate top priority. By keeping these and other important considerations in mind, the collaborative group is likely to develop an action plan that is realistic and well conceived.

The group will need to clarify roles in the change process. The collaborative group should assess and then effectively utilize the talents and expertise of its members. Typically, there is much work to do and the group can distribute responsibilities to all group members without overburdening one person. This is one of many advantages of working with a group. As the group assesses the talents and expertise of members, it should not overlook the specific expertise of the school counselor trained as a leader and advocate. The school counselor should be a likely candidate for coordinating the advocacy-for-change efforts. The counselor is trained to work effectively with all departments within a school and a school district.

The group will need to collect data to monitor the impact of action steps and progress toward objectives. Stakeholders will seek accountability from the change agents. Disaggregation of data by demographics such as race, gender, and socioeconomic status as well as other relevant factors is necessary to sort out the impact of action plans on the status of various groups of students.

A clear and detailed timeline that includes specific action steps serves as a visual representation of the change agenda and a document that can be used to promote accountability. The collaborative group can utilize the timeline to monitor progress on the change agenda, noting and celebrating successes along the way. The timeline can make the group aware of obstacles along the way and alert the group of the need for more intensified or alternative advocacy strategies.

Step 9: Identify Policies/Practices That Need to Change, and Develop Change Strategies

In order to identify the policies and practices that present barriers to necessary systemic change, the collaborative change group can consider the following questions: Which policies and practices interfere with the goals and objectives of the proposed systemic change? What can the group do to address these policies and practices and eliminate the barriers they cause? The resulting strategies should keep the change agenda on course.

Step 10: Enlist the Support of Influential People and Policy Makers

In order to strengthen the power of the change efforts, the collaborative group must identify and enlist the support of influential people and policy makers. This may include leaders of parents' and teachers' organizations, curriculum specialists, administrators, school board members, legislators, social justice organizations, organizations for educational reform, and various other local and national community leaders.

Step 11: Identify and Challenge Resistance

Advocates/change agents must act with a sense of empowerment when challenging sources of resistance and opposition. They are more effective when they work in groups. There is power in working together in groups rather than as lone activists in isolation. Another way to enhance power in advocacy efforts is to keep change efforts visible. The collaborative group can appear in the various media, invite community involvement, and create political pressure.

Step 12: Evaluate Progress and Revise the Plan as Needed

In order to evaluate progress, the collaborative group must identify indicators of success. Group members must reach a consensus on the criteria for success with the change agenda. They must identify and specify success indicators so that they are easy to measure. It is useful to identify the indicators that demonstrate immediate and direct benefits to students, for example, students are safer in their school, in addition to indicators that reflect an impact on the system and, ultimately, on students, for example, revised policies and procedures.

Step 13: Share the Results

Following student advocacy efforts using the Education Trust Advocacy Model, it is important to share the results with stakeholders and decision makers. This may include principals, superintendents, the school board, parents, students, teachers, the community, and others. When sharing data, it is helpful to create an effective presentation using visual aids such as bar and line graphs and pie charts and other information such as lists of trends from data and individualized stories without identifying information. Often, when a group shares data in this manner, the audience may raise questions that will require additional study and data collection. As this process unfolds, more stakeholders become participants in leadership and advocacy efforts.

Self-Assessment and Exploration

In this exercise, you contact a professional school counselor or school administrator to review the approach to a problem in a school setting. Explain the assignment. Address the thirteen steps of the Education Trust advocacy approach. Reviewing the model with a real-life problem situation makes for a more meaningful learning process. If possible, use this process with your supervisor's permission during internship.

Instructions: Complete the following worksheet and share a copy with the counselor or administrator if it would be of use to them.

A. Preliminary Steps

1. Identify the problem and the extent of the problem using data.

_____

_____

_____

_____

2. Determine systemic contributions to the problem.

_____

_____

_____

_____

3. Assess the risks of action versus inaction.

_____

_____

_____

_____

4. Identify allies.

_____

_____

_____

_____

_____

5. Identify opportunities to address the problem through teaming and collaboration.

_____

_____

_____

_____

_____

6. Work with allies to clarify the source and focus of the problem.

_____

_____

_____

_____

_____

7. Gather additional data to support the need for change.

_____

_____

_____

_____

_____

B. Action Steps

8. Delineate an action plan and take only realistic action.

_____

_____

_____

_____

_____

9. Identify policies/practices that need to change and develop change strategies.

_____

_____

_____

_____

_____

10. Enlist the support of influential people and policy makers.

_____

_____

_____

_____

_____

11. Identify sources of resistance and develop strategies for addressing/challenging it.

_____

_____

_____

_____

_____

12. Evaluate progress and revise the plan as needed.

_____

_____

_____

_____

_____

13. Share the results.

_____

_____

_____

_____

_____

Overriding Principles

The Education Trust (2002) identified the following eight overriding principles, which are recommended when school counselors advocate for systems change:

1. Act with purpose.
2. Act ethically.
3. Keep lines of communication open.
4. Keep efforts visible.
5. Remain hopeful.
6. Think ahead.
7. Work collaboratively.
8. Remember: Advocating for change is a long process.

CHAPTER SUMMARY

School counselors serve as advocates when they assertively argue a cause on behalf of their students, schools, and their profession. Effective advocacy frequently requires collaboration, in which a group of people work together toward a common goal. The focus is on relationships that enrich the process of goal achievement and involves pooling the resources of a diverse group of stakeholders that mirrors the characteristics of the school and local community. Collaboration is a voluntary process.

In our rapidly changing and increasingly diverse society with its many pressures on schools and students, the mandate for school counselor advocacy for children, school personnel, schools, districts, and the school counseling profession is great and nonnegotiable. The Education Trust offers school counselor advocates a 13-step model of advocacy that incorporates principles of effective educational leadership. Guiding the advocacy process are eight overriding principles that remind the advocate to act purposefully and ethically, communicate openly and continuously while keeping one's efforts visible, remain hopeful and think ahead, and collaborate and be patient while keeping in mind the long process involved in effecting change.

REVIEW AND REFLECT

1. From the list that follows or your own ideas, identify and prioritize three of the most common advocacy issues you believe you are likely to encounter in your work as a school counselor. What are you doing now as a new-vision counselor to prepare to face and address these issues?

   ____ racial prejudice

   ____ high dropout rates

   ____ difficulties accessing college

   ____ bullying

   ____ achievement gaps

   ____ poor attendance

   ____ low standardized test scores

_____ underperforming students

_____ other _____

The instructor or a classmate should write the list on a chalk- or whiteboard and tally the class's responses. In a class discussion, share your rationale for your responses.

2. Do an Internet search for articles on advocacy issues in schools. Review titles and abstracts and choose two relevant articles to read. How can you utilize what you learned from these readings in your own advocacy project in the school where you intern or work? Summarize key findings with your learning group. These summaries could also be posted on an electronic discussion board.

RELEVANT WEBSITES

American Association of School Administrators: www.aasa.org/

American School Counselor Association: www.schoolcounselor.org

Association for Supervision and Curriculum Development: www.ascd.org

Eye on Education: www.eyeoneducation.com

National Association of Secondary School Principals:
www.principals.org/www.questia.com/

Reviews of educational policies and practices effective in closing the achievement gap: www.ed.gov/databases/ERIC_Digests/ed460191.html

Richard Cohen Films: www.richardcohenfilms.com

The College Board: www.collegeboard.com

The Education Trust: www.edtrust.org

The International Center for Leadership in Education: www.daggett.com/

The National Association for College Admissions Counseling:
www.info@nacac.com

The School Leadership Development Unit: www.sofweb.vic.edu.au/pd/schlead/
http://21stcenturyschools.northcarolina.edu/center

REFERENCES

Anderson, B., Fortson, B. W., IV, Kleinedler, S. R., & Schonthal, H. (Eds.). (2001). *American Heritage Dictionary* (4th ed.). Boston: Houghton Mifflin Company.

Baker, S. B., & Gerler, E. R., Jr. (2004). *School counseling for the twenty-first century.* Upper Saddle River, NJ: Merrill Prentice Hall.

Bolman, L., & Deal, T. (1994). *Becoming a teacher leader: From isolation to collaboration.* Thousand Oaks, CA: Corwin Press.

Council for Accreditation of Counseling and Related Educational Programs. (1999, September). *2001 CACREP accreditation standards and procedures manual* (Draft 3). Alexandria, VA: Author.

Education Trust. (1999). *Transforming school counseling initiative* [Brochure]. Washington, DC: Author.

Education Trust. (2002). *National school counselor training initiative* [Brochure]. Jacksonville, FL: Author.

Education Trust. (2003). *National school counselor training initiative* (Rev. ed.) [Brochure]. Jacksonville, FL: Author.

Eldridge, W. D. (1983). Affirmative small social action and the use of power in clinical counseling. *Counseling and Values, 27*, 66–77.

Homan, M. S. (1999). *Promoting community change: Making it happen in the real world* (2nd ed.). Pacific Grove, CA: Brooks/Cole.

Lee, C., & Walz, G. R. (Eds.). (1998). *Social action: A mandate for counselors.* Alexandria, VA: American Counseling Association.

Menacker, J. (1976). Toward a theory of activist guidance. *Personnel and Guidance Journal, 54*, 318–321.

Ponzo, Z. (1974). A counselor and change: Reminiscences and resolution. *Personnel and Guidance Journal, 53*, 27–32.

CHAPTER 10
Leadership in Collaboration and Consultation

A DEMONSTRATION OF THE POWER OF COLLABORATION

The parents and teachers of Morton Elementary School recently learned that their school counselor's position was going to be cut due to budgetary limits. Under pressure from the district administration on one side and the school's parent-teacher organization on the other, the newly-hired principal worked out a plan with the district administration to share a counselor from a nearby elementary school. The counselor would work at the Morton school one and a half days a week. The principal hoped that would satisfy all parties involved.

Maureen, a school counselor, had worked full time at Morton Elementary School for three years and had been hired with federal elementary school demonstration grant monies. She had become well acquainted with the children, the teachers, the administrators, other staff, and parents and had collaborated with many of them on various school committees. She had developed a comprehensive, competency-based school counseling program in which she focused on meeting the needs of all children in the school. Although her comprehensive school guidance program was fairly new and she needed some time to demonstrate its effectiveness on academic achievement, she already had collected preliminary data showing its positive impact on student performance, including reading performance.

Both the principal and district administration had intended to include funds in the budget to keep the school counselor. However, based on No Child Left Behind standards, the school was designated as underperforming, and the school improvement team had recommended that the school hire a reading specialist to help increase the reading performance of the students. This recommendation created pressure on the principal to comply with the district administration's plan. Meanwhile, the school counselor compiled and shared a report with the principal, school improvement team, and parents, including her promising data from the school and the results of national school counselor research that indicated the positive influence of guidance activities on academic achievement (Whiston & Sexton, 1998; Wilson, 1986) and improved academic achievement of students who receive counseling (Borders & Drury, 1992).

Case Discussion

Questions About This Case

- What were some of the key issues that this school counselor faced?
- What other options did she have for responding to the challenges she faced?
- How can school collaborators support the mission of school counselors?
- What messages about school counselor roles and priorities does this scenario convey?
- What can we learn from this case example about working with the stakeholders in a school?

Further Thoughts on This Case

In the situation at the Morton Elementary School, parents and teachers expressed strong opposition to the plan of cutting the counselor's position and hiring a reading specialist. Maureen had educated them about the research support for guidance programs, and many of them had observed firsthand the benefits of the school counselor's presence and the comprehensive school counseling program's impact on the personal and academic skills of their children. They believed that their children's standardized test scores did not yet reflect the extent of their actual gains. A group of parents and teachers who Maureen had trained in advocacy procedures met several times, did some research on reading achievement to add to materials previously compiled, and proposed an alternative plan to improve their children's standardized reading scores by including the counselor, administration, teachers, parents, grandparents, and community volunteers in a program that stressed reading and improved preparation for the standardized test. The teachers, counselor, and parents had the previous principal's support for starting the alternative reading program this school year. The whole-school approach to reading improvement included a guidance curriculum that strongly supported its objectives.

The parents contacted the local newspaper and convinced it to have a reporter do a feature article about the school's triumphs and challenges and its collaborative advocacy effort to retain the comprehensive guidance program. As a result of the article, they received overwhelming support from the community including letters of support for the counselor and the comprehensive guidance program to the superintendent, the school board, the principal, and the editor of the local newspaper, encouraging phone calls, donations of reading materials, money, and volunteer time dedicated to the alternative reading program. Maureen's history of successful collaboration in the interest of the needs of her students laid the foundation for a strong collaborative effort of the school stakeholders to support her and the comprehensive school counseling program focused on academic success that she had put in place.

CHAPTER OBJECTIVES

The objectives of this chapter are to:

1. Outline the principles of effective educational collaboration.
2. Identify targets of and resources for collaborative efforts within the school system.

WHAT COLLABORATION IS AND WHY IT IS NECESSARY

The example at the beginning of this chapter illustrates the power inherent in collaborative relationships with a common vision. It also illustrates the empowering nature of shared leadership of a common cause for the individuals involved. Collaboration is a necessary part of a school counselor's job (Porter, Epp, & Bryant, 2000). The Education Trust (2002) developed a position statement on teaming and collaboration for school counselors. The first part of that statement follows.

> The new vision for school counseling, developed as part of the Transforming School Counseling Initiative, calls for the school counselors to extend their traditional responsibilities to embrace roles as educational leaders, team-builders and collaborators, advocates, and users of assessment data in order to enhance educational experiences and outcomes for all students.

This chapter outlines principles of effective teaming, collaboration, and consultation for school counselors and identifies targets and resources for school counselors' efforts in those areas.

PRINCIPLES OF EFFECTIVE TEAMING, COLLABORATION, AND CONSULTATION

Friend and Cook (1996) explain interpersonal collaboration as "a style for direct interaction between at least two coequal parties voluntarily engaged in shared decision making as they work toward a common goal" (p. 6). Collaboration is one type of interactive process that can be used to accomplish a goal. The word *collaboration* implies that those collaborating have a common goal.

Friend and Cook (1996) identified defining characteristics of collaboration: voluntary, parity of participants, based on mutual goals, shared responsibility for participation and decision making, shared resources, and shared accountability for outcomes. People who collaborate typically value the collaboration, trust other people, and gain a sense of community from the process. Collaboration is a trend currently being promoted in educational leadership training and educational reform.

Collaborative groups can accomplish tasks that would be difficult or impossible for an individual to accomplish. They generally have more power to change systems than individual efforts. The collaborative approach tends to create a common language and better understanding of issues affecting students and academic achievement within a school or a district. Collaboration can lead to the development of networks of comprehensive services for children and adolescents. The approach provides a way to engage key stakeholders regarding issues of concern. Collaboration leads to the development of a greater sense of community in the collaborators.

The Education Trust (2002) emphasized the need for school counselors to be team builders and collaborators. School counselors need to work with teachers, administrators, staff, students, family members, and the community in service of the school's mission. School counselors receive training in group dynamics and group processes that prepares them for teamwork and collaboration. Azar (1997) defined *team* as a group of "two or more people who interact dynamically, interdependently, and adaptively and who share at least one common goal or purpose" (p. 14).

Leadership in Collaboration

Lao Tzu's thoughts on leadership in collaborative groups are quoted by Heider (1986):

> What we call leadership consists mainly of knowing how to follow. The wise leader stays in the background and facilitates other people's process. The greatest things the leader does go largely unnoticed. Because the leader does not push or shape or manipulate, there is no resentment or resistance (p. 131).

Some of the components of a productive team process, described by Johnson and Johnson (2000), include: shared leadership responsibilities, well-defined and well-understood purpose, mission and goals, effectiveness measured by outcomes and products, accountability of members and the group, time for interaction and celebration of individual and group success, content and process needs to be monitored, clear ground rules, reasonable and attainable goals, continued processing of team effectiveness, and ways to improve. School counselors can foster team building and collaboration by consciously incorporating these components in their work.

Leadership in Consultation

When referring to the work of school counselors, the term collaboration is often seen in conjunction with consultation. When a school counselor serves as a consultant, he/she works with a person or group of people (consultee/consultees) with the goal of influencing change in someone else, usually a child. The school counselor consultant is systems oriented and helps those involved to conceptualize a problem in the context of the bigger picture. Typically, the school counselor consults with parents, teachers, and other school personnel regarding students.

Satisfying consultative relationships that focus on student behavior and performance can lead to effective collaborative relationships. Keys, Bemak, Carpenter, and King-Sears (1998) described a collaborative consultative model for addressing the complicated problems of children and families today. They offer a five-stage problem-solving collaborative consultation model: coming together to obtain commitment to collaborate, identifying a shared vision, developing an action plan for goals and objectives, implementing the action plan, and evaluating progress.

The School Counselor as Relationship Builder

In the book *Leadership*, Dubrin (2004) identifies seven relationship-oriented attitudes and behaviors that help to get people working together smoothly. They include:

1. Aligning and mobilizing people—getting people to work together smoothly.
2. Concert building—building a work group into a well-functioning, ongoing system.
3. Creating inspiration—triggering powerful emotional experiences in others by building enthusiasm, stimulating thinking, enabling leadership in others, recognizing others' contributions, and developing people's talents. Being visible and accessible reinforces inspiration.
4. Satisfying higher-level needs—learning what is important to others and facilitating opportunities for getting those needs met.
5. Giving emotional support and encouragement—accomplished by expressing appreciation of others and through the sharing of leadership and decision-making opportunities.
6. Promoting principles and values—advocating for good causes uplifts and motivates others to care about and act in the interest of the common good.
7. Being a servant leader—being committed to service and helping others achieve their goals.

Self-Assessment and Exploration

In this exercise, you will rate your relationship-oriented attitudes and behaviors.

A.   Rate yourself on a scale of 1 to 5 on these seven attitudes and behaviors as described by Dubrin (2004). (1 = very weak, 5 = very strong)

Relationship-Oriented Attitudes and Behaviors	Very Weak ⟵ ⟶ Very Strong				
Aligning and mobilizing people	1	2	3	4	5
Concert building	1	2	3	4	5
Creating inspiration	1	2	3	4	5
Satisfying higher-level needs	1	2	3	4	5
Giving emotional support and encouragement	1	2	3	4	5
Promoting principles and values	1	2	3	4	5
Being a servant leader	1	2	3	4	5

B. Look at your scores on each of the leadership relationship dimensions. Consider the categories you scored at 4 or 5, strengths, and those you scored at 1 or 2, areas for improvement. Make note of your strengths and areas for improvement. Consider the areas listed for improvement when you review and revise your leadership improvement plan.

A COLLABORATIVE MODEL IN PRACTICE

An example of university-school district collaboration can be explored through this framework. Several years ago, as a new school counselor educator, one of the authors (DeVoss) sought to develop a collaborative team/advisory council for the school counseling program that she coordinated. She sought out other stakeholders who were interested in the preparation of school counselors. Prospective members of the advisory council were sought who would be able to enrich discussions, contribute to goal setting and problem solving in the university school counseling program, collaborate with university faculty to continuously improve school counselor preparation.

Through networking while attending various university and school district meetings, potential collaborators emerged. An adjunct professor in the educational leadership department of the authors' university, who was a retired school counselor, agreed to teach in the school counseling program and be on the program's advisory council. Two coordinators of the guidance program for the largest school district in the area expressed strong interest in ensuring that the program met national and state standards and the needs of local school districts. A professor in the educational psychology department where the program is housed was interested in assuring that the program attracted and retained qualified minority students and promoted multicultural competencies in the school counselor trainees. A currently practicing school counselor who also worked in private practice was interested in establishing high standards of clinical training for the counseling students. These were the initial core collaborators in the school counseling master's of education program.

As noted, the collaborators were identified through networking in professional meetings. The group came together by invitation to meetings at the university to discuss the school counseling program. At these meetings, all participants committed to collaborate on the issue of high-quality school counselor preparation. Using guidelines of the Educational Trust as a model, the group discussed and defined a shared vision of educational equity in a culturally diverse society. The collaborators discussed a shared vision of school counseling in the 21st century and developed a document that outlined the program's mission statement and commitments to strengthen the program and develop it to be more sensitive and responsive to the needs of K–12 schools and students in the 21st century.

The group built trust as members worked collaboratively. Group members reported genuine enjoyment of the collegial atmosphere and the common goals on which everyone was focused. The collaborative group determined goals and objectives by using the Educational Trust's eight essential elements for transforming school counseling as guidelines and adding ideas from members' own backgrounds and experiences. The strategic plan to accomplish goals and objectives was a detailed document based on the eight essential elements. This document identified the timeline and the responsible party for each plan of action. The group decided that the evaluation of progress on goals and specific objectives would be based on evidence that specific actions had taken place and the degree to which goals and objectives were accomplished (for example, selection process to use multiple criteria reflecting the values in the mission statement and the overall percentage and percentage increase in minority students in newly recruited cohorts to demonstrate commitment to the recruitment of minorities). The strategic plan document specified the data to be collected for each objective.

PREPARING TO DEVELOP A COLLABORATIVE TEAM

In keeping with the ASCA National Model (2003), collaborative efforts in schools need to be data driven. In other words, collaborators come together to address concerns reflected in school data (for example, graduation and dropout rates, failure rates in specific classes, attendance information, percentages of various racial/ethnic/SES groups in AP classes, incidents of bullying). The data provide a common ground and starting point for a group of collaborators who potentially come from diverse backgrounds. The following series of questions provides a set of guidelines for developing a collaborative team.

1. Who are potential team members and collaborators with similar goals and values?
2. How will the collaborators "come together"?
3. How will all participants establish commitment to collaborate on an issue of common concern?
4. How will the collaborators go about defining a shared vision?
5. What ideas, information, and knowledge would the team like to include in the vision?
6. How will team members build trust as collaborators?
7. How will the collaborators determine goals and objectives?
8. What ideas for goals and objectives will the collaborators bring to the table?
9. What will the strategic plan to accomplish goals and objectives look like?
10. Who will do what on the action plan?
11. What is the timeline for implementation of the plan?
12. How will progress on goals and specific objectives be evaluated?
13. What type of data will be collected to demonstrate progress?

Adapted from Keys, Bemak, Carpenter, and King-Sears (1998) and the Education Trust (2002).

CHAPTER SUMMARY

School counselors can learn to be effective collaborators by using principles of effective educational collaboration such as aligning and mobilizing people, concert building, creating inspiration, employing servant leadership, and others reviewed in this chapter. In addition, they can proactively identify targets for collaborative efforts within the school system as well as the resources needed and available for those efforts. School counselors can tap into the power inherent in collaborative relationships with a common vision to benefit students. They can prepare for the development of collaborative teams by reviewing the guiding questions provided by the collaborative consultation model developed by Keys, Bemak, Carpenter, and King-Sears (1998).

REVIEW AND REFLECT

Use the Keys, Bemak, Carpenter, and King-Sears (1998) collaborative consultation model to describe how you might approach a problem like Maureen's in the case at the beginning of the chapter. You are not expected to actually carry out the process but only to reflect on each of the steps. If you prefer, you can use a school-related problem in which you currently have an investment. Or, you can use one of the issues examined in the Review and Reflect exercise on advocacy in Chapter 9. Consider how you might accomplish the five steps of the model. Make notes to share in a small- or large-group discussion.

Issue to be examined: _____

1. Who will your collaborators be? How will you "come together"? How will you establish the commitment of all participants to collaborate on a certain issue?

_____

_____

_____

_____

_____

_____

_____

_____

_____

2. How will you go about defining a shared vision? What are some of the ideas, information, and knowledge you would like to include in the vision? How will you build trust with your collaborators? How will you determine goals and objectives? What ideas for goals and objectives will you bring to the table?

_____

_____

_____

_____

_____

_____

_____

_____

_____

3. Imagine what the strategic plan to accomplish goals and objectives might look like. Who will do what on the action plan? What is the timeline for implementation of the plan?

_____

_____

_____

_____

_____

_____

_____

_____

_____

_____

4. How will progress on goals and specific objectives be evaluated? What type of data will be collected to demonstrate progress?

_____

_____

_____

_____

_____

_____

_____

_____

RELEVANT WEBSITES

American School Counselor Association: www.schoolcounselor.org

Eye on Education: www.eyeoneducation.com

Reviews of educational policies and practices effective in closing the achievement gap: www.ed.gov/databases/ERIC_Digests/ed460191.html

The Education Trust: www.edtrust.org

The International Center for Leadership in Education: www.daggett.com/

The School Leadership Development Unit: www.sofweb.vic.edu.au/pd/schlead/ http://21stcenturyschools.northcarolina.edu/center

REFERENCES

Azar, B. (1997, July). Teambuilding isn't enough: Workers need training too. *APA Monitor, 28*(7), 1–16.

Baker, S. B., & Gerler, E. R., Jr. (2004). *School counseling for the twenty-first century.* Upper Saddle River, NJ: Pearson Education, Inc.

Borders, L., & Drury, S. (1992). Comprehensive school counseling programs: A review for policymakers and practitioners. *Journal of Counseling and Development, 70,* 487–498.

Dubrin, A. J. (2004). *Leadership: Research findings, practice, and skills.* Boston: Houghton Mifflin Company.

Education Trust. (2002). *National school counselor training initiative* [Brochure]. Jacksonville, FL: Author.

Friend, M., & Cook, L., (1996). *Interactions: Collaboration skills for school professionals* (2nd ed.). White Plains, NY: Longman Publishers.

Heider, J. (1986) *The tao of leadership.* New York: Bantam Books.

Keys, S., Bemak, F., Carpenter, S., & King-Sears, M. (1998). Collaborative consultant: A new role for counselors serving at-risk youth. *Journal of Counseling and Development, 76,* 123–133.

Johnson, D. W., and Johnson, F. P. (2000). *Joining together.* Boston: Allyn & Bacon.

Porter, G., Epp, L., & Bryant, S. (2000). Collaboration among school mental health professionals: A necessity, not a luxury. *Professional School Counseling, 3,* 315–322.

Whiston, S., & Sexton, T. (1998). A review of school counseling outcome research: Implications for practice. *Journal of Counseling and Development, 76,* 412–426.

Wilson, N. S. (1986). Effects of a classroom guidance unit on sixth graders' examination performance. *Journal of Humanistic Education and Development, 25*(2), 70–79.

CHAPTER 11

Leadership, Accountability, and Data

A COUNSELOR'S SPOTLIGHT ON OPPORTUNITY

During her counseling internship, Lynn learned that very few of the students at her field placement high school were taking advantage of a program offering services and financial assistance at the local community college. Although many students planned to attend the community college and were eligible for the Achieving a College Education program (ACE), few students at Marana High School (only two in the previous spring) applied to the program.

The ACE program was cosponsored by the local community college and the university. ACE provided financial assistance, guidance, advisement, and career exploration to the average hardworking student. Based on the information Lynn had, she identified this situation as an opportunity for change within the school. She identified the resources needed to facilitate systems change in Marana High School: students, parents, teachers, counselors, the community college, and the university. She worked with the groups and institutions identified and developed an objective of increasing the number of students in the ACE program from Marana High School. Lynn believed that by accomplishing this task, the school would facilitate access to higher education for average hardworking students who might not otherwise attend college.

Early in the spring 2004 semester, Lynn learned as much as possible about the ACE program. She then disseminated information to all 10th graders through teacher-approved classroom presentations in all English composition classes. Students signed up if they thought they could qualify for the ACE program based on class rank and GPA guidelines provided to them. Lynn followed up with the students who thought they could qualify by distributing 80 applications and informing students when the applications were due and that she was available to assist them. The applications were due in early April. By the end of the spring 2004 semester, 15 students asked for assistance in completing the application and 13 actually completed them.

Lynn compared the number of students who applied for the ACE program the year she intervened (13) to the previous year (2) and the number of students who were accepted during the year she intervened (11) to the number accepted in the previous year (1). In addition, she located data on the total number of students who had applied to ACE in the past and the total number who had been accepted and enrolled in ACE. She planned to find out how many ACE students from Marana High School and all area high schools completed either associate's or bachelor's degrees.

Another school counselor, Maria, recently hired at another high school, noticed that a large number of seniors at her college-preparatory school were not prepared for the college application process. She observed many seniors beginning their senior school year without a clear idea of what was needed for the college application process. She decided to call on the resources of students, parents, colleges, her school's college counselor, teachers, and class counselors to assist in systems change that would prepare students in her high school for the college application process before their senior year. Students would have the necessary information available and be prepared to use it.

Maria assisted the other counselors in becoming acquainted with the Arizona mentor program software. She prepared all counselors to assist their advisees in setting up their own accounts. All of the school's counselors became proficient in the software by the end of April of the first year and began implementation with students in the fall of that year. The system was to be in place so that the graduating classes of three and four years later could be familiar with the software and effectively use their accounts and be prepared for the college application process before their senior year.

Maria planned ongoing evaluation of the effectiveness of incorporating the software program through pretests and posttests. In addition, she distributed surveys to the school counselors to assess their opinions of the software and its usefulness.

Case Discussion

Questions About This Case

- In what ways did these school counseling interns use leadership skills?
- What was the impact on the system of the interventions made by these interns?
- How can school counseling interventions such as these support the mission of the school?
- What messages about school counselor roles and priorities does this scenario convey?
- What can we learn from this case example about working with others in a school?

Further Thoughts on This Case

Lynn and Maria are excellent examples of new school counselors who are becoming proficient at using data to drive school counselor interventions on behalf of their students. Although new in the profession, they have quickly earned the respect of more experienced school counselors who have observed their use of data to initiate systemic change in their schools. They used their leadership skills effectively to obtain support and encouragement from their departments, administration, students, and parents to advocate for students.

CHAPTER OBJECTIVES

The objectives of this chapter are to:

1. Provide the rationale for school counselors to collect and analyze data relevant to school counseling programs.
2. Provide guidelines for developing data-driven comprehensive school counseling programs.

DATA-DRIVEN SCHOOL COUNSELING PROGRAMS

Why are data so important? More specifically, why are data so important to school counselors as educational leaders? Don't they have enough to do already without having to work with data? We know that school counselors have many demands on their time. Why not allow them to just keep doing all the excellent work they have been doing, helping students and supporting the mission of schools? Why add even one more thing to their already full plates?

Schools are in the midst of reform efforts. It is educational data that has sparked these reforms. Data have informed educators that we have not been providing high-quality education to all students and we have not ensured that all students have equal access to postsecondary education. There continues to be an achievement gap between poor and minority students and students from the dominant culture. This educational achievement gap leads to inequities in opportunities for success for the lower-achieving groups. Traditionally, school counselors have not been known for demonstrating accountability. By collecting and presenting data that connect the school guidance program with academic achievement, they can demonstrate both accountability and leadership. Today, school counselors as educational leaders recognize the importance of having a voice in educational reform. They realize that creating a voice begins by demonstrating accountability through school counseling program data.

The Power in Data

Data speak loudly. They create a sense of urgency. They cry out for change and for deliberate and focused action plans. Data catch the attention of educational leaders and decision makers who are held accountable for educational results represented by the data. Data provide evidence when there are inequities and lack of access, and data create a mandate for social change. As a plan for change is put into place, the collection of data serves to monitor progress and indicates where adjustments in the plan may be necessary. Data are required when requesting funding for programming to support systems change.

It is necessary to disaggregate data by race and gender to identify specific areas of inequity or lack of access. Types of data that are important to collect include: attendance rates, dropout rates, graduation rates, college acceptance rates, college attendance rates, rates of completion of homework, failure rates, incidents of bullying or violence, and rates of English proficiency. Most of this type of data is available through the school district data system. School counselors generally have easy access to the data and need only to become familiar with the data system to have current data at their fingertips.

With No Child Left Behind (NCLB) a reality, this is an age of accountability and high-stakes testing. Teachers and administrators feel the pressure of their jobs on the line based on student standardized test scores. School counselors traditionally were left out of school reform efforts. Things have changed recently, however: School counselors have now become active leaders and team members for school reform. Like students, parents, teachers, and administrators, school counselors are also concerned about the impact of standardized testing on the school system.

As educational leaders, school counselors must be accountable. They must demonstrate their contribution to student achievement. The ASCA *National Model* (2003) section on accountability asks the question, "How are students different as a result of the school counseling program?" (p. 23). School counselors are expected to answer this question with evidence from their school's data. They need the feedback the data provide in order to determine whether what they are doing is working or whether another approach is in order. Schmidt (2003) stated, "The future credibility and efficacy of the profession depend on counselors taking the lead and demonstrating their value to the school community and to the educational process" (p. 241).

School Counselor Accountability

School counselors are increasingly being expected to account for their contributions to student achievement. School decision makers are interested in how children are better off from having a school counselor in their school. In addition to this push for accountability there is an ethical responsibility for school counselors to make informed decisions about counseling interventions based on data.

Schmidt (2003) stated that school counseling program goals must be agreed upon by those involved in evaluating the outcomes and understood and accepted by those involved in the program. The evaluation process should include everyone served by the school counseling program. Instrumentation and evaluation processes should be valid for the purposes for which they are used. Evaluation of the school counseling program is a continuous process built in to the comprehensive school counseling program starting with the development phase. School counselors need strong leadership and support from state and local educational leaders in order to build and maintain comprehensive school counseling programs with an ongoing accountability component.

As part of their accountability, school counselors participate in their own performance appraisal, which determines how the counselor and the school counseling program have contributed to the mission of the school. School counselor performance appraisals highlight the counselor's strengths and areas that need improvement. Counselor appraisals also provide information to guide decisions about professional development needs.

The program evaluation and counselor appraisal processes are part of a continuous feedback loop in which counselors have the opportunity to plan change and implement adjustments based on what they learn about the program and their professional skills. For greatest effectiveness, program evaluation and counselor appraisal need to provide a balanced perspective, including both positive and negative feedback (Schmidt, 2003; Atkinson, Furlong, & Janoff, 1979; Fairchild, 1986; Gysbers, Lapan, & Blair, 1999; Krumboltz, 1974).

Self-Assessment and Exploration

In this exercise you will explore the role of research in school counselor accountability.

A. Review recent editions of *The Professional School Counselor* and select a research article written by a practicing school counselor (not a counselor educator). Write a brief summary of the article for your learning group. Post it online if there is a bulletin board or discussion location for your class or e-mail an attachment to your learning group.

B. Reflect on the following questions regarding the article and yourself as you consider incorporating research activities into your own practice as a school counselor:

1. How relevant to daily school counseling practice was the study in the article?

_____

_____

_____

_____

_____

2. Was the methodology used in the study clear, and was the study one that you could replicate?

_____

_____

_____

_____

3. What questions about school counseling do you think should be answered through research?

_____

_____

_____

_____

_____

4. What type of research is most useful to school counselors? (This might involve some investigation.)

_____

_____

_____

_____

_____

5. On a scale of 0 to 10, how comfortable do you feel with the incorporation of research activities into your practice as a school counselor?

Not at all comfortable $\longleftarrow$ —————— $\longrightarrow$ Completely comfortable

0   1   2   3   4   5   6   7   8   9   10

6. If your score was 5 or lower, what would it take for you to feel more comfortable and/or competent? Share your responses to these questions with a learning partner.

_____

_____

_____

_____

_____

Types of Data

Most school counselors work with data in the form of standardized test results. This is generally familiar territory. Counselors become familiar with standardized educational tests during their master's degree training. School counselors frequently play a key role in their school's standardized testing program. They are often involved in administering tests and, later, in interpreting the results for students and parents. School counselors may help students use their test scores to choose specific career paths and preparation courses as well as to make plans for postsecondary education.

The same familiar test scores that measure academic achievement can be utilized as a source of outcome data indicating the effectiveness of school counseling interventions. However, it is important to use multiple sources of outcome data. School counselors typically include other sources of data, such as teacher and parent ratings, observations, checklists, and their own documented observations of students. Pretests and posttests can be especially useful in documenting changes in student behavior before and after specific counseling interventions.

In development of the school counseling program, the school counselor needs to consciously consider existing school and district data in disaggregated form. This allows the counselor to identify the gaps in learning from one group of students to another. The counselor can then provide a rationale for the need for change and propose appropriate interventions that promote academic achievement for all students.

Working with Data

This section provides guidelines for school counselors' use of data in the course of their daily work. It offers a starting place and a systematic approach to incorporating data utilization in developing, maintaining, and evaluating school counseling programs. The guidelines include becoming familiar with the school district's data system, analyzing disaggregated data to identify achievement gaps among groups of students, identifying areas for targeted change, designing interventions to bring about the desired change, and evaluating outcomes. Of course, to maximize effectiveness, the school counselor should engage others in these processes. The school and district's focus on providing a good education to all students is shared by school counselors and school administrators, teachers, staff, colleagues, parents, and the counseling program's advisory council.

Getting to Know the Data

One of the new school counselor's first tasks should be to become familiar with the data collection system of his/her school. This typically translates into logging on to the school district's database and locating the types of data being collected by the district and individual schools. The counselor should learn how to locate student-achievement data that indicate academic progress. Examples of achievement data include dropout rates, grade point averages, standardized test data, and graduation rates. Related data include discipline and suspension incidents, attendance and tardiness rates, and completion-of-homework rates. The school counselor may require some basic training to become competent at navigating the database.

Another source of outcome data is measures of student mastery of the ASCA National Model competencies such as the percentage of students who apply time-management and task-management skills (A:A2), maintain a career-planning portfolio (C:B2.5), or identify personal strengths and assets (PS:A1.10). This type of data demonstrates the school counseling program's progress in providing comprehensive guidance services to all students.

An important activity involving relevant data for school counselors is analyzing disaggregated data from the district's data system to identify achievement gaps among groups of students. This has the effect of looking at educational data under a microscope. When examining school data this closely, school counselors will find inequities among groups, creating the opportunity to develop a focused agenda with specific targets for change that are based on the data.

LEADERSHIP: ROCKING THE BOAT WITH DATA

An agenda for change typically involves change at the systems level. This kind of change will disrupt the status quo. It will interrupt "business as usual" in the school. There will likely be resistance from various quarters. The school counselor who is trained as a leader and advocate will be ready for resistance with a toolbox of approaches for handling it.

Some of those tools include recruiting powerful people who support the agenda for change and some of the likely resisters to change to serve on the change committee. The data can be used to logically support the proposed change. The data can speak for themselves and identify areas for targeted change based on clearly documented inequities. Data can be used to maintain a high profile for the change effort, with regular progress updates to stakeholders. By sharing the work, the counselor and the change committee can share the investment in change and the sense of empowerment that accompanies working as change agents. Working as a group allows you to maximize the leadership strengths of the various group members.

Benchmarking and Total Quality Improvement

In this age of educational reform, there are schools that have become exemplary in their organizational practices. Other schools can learn from these schools through a systematic process that originated with the Total Quality Improvement approach known as benchmarking (Tucker, 1996). Benchmarking is a process whereby one school that needs to improve in a particular area learns from a high-performing school by comparing the performance of one to the other. It is an involved process that takes time and patience, and requires reserving judgment while performing as objective a comparison as possible of one school to the other. The goal is learning and adapting what one learns to the specific needs of the school in need of change.

The benchmarking process involves studying all contributions to the outcomes of the exemplary school. It is based on a systems approach to quality improvement and involves the examining organizational strategies, programs, processes, and procedures. The school using benchmarking needs to make a major commitment of time and energy in order to do it well. It is not meant to be a process in which one school copies the practices of another school. Benchmarking can be an opportunity for school counselors and other educational leaders to collaborate with parents and other stakeholders on behalf of school improvement.

The school that utilizes benchmarking must start by studying its own operation and asking questions about what it is doing, how it is doing it, and how well it is doing it. The school will ask the same questions about the exemplary school it is studying for comparison. In addition, the school doing the study must ask why it gets the results it gets as opposed to the results of the school being studied. Throughout the benchmarking process, the school improvement team must keep in mind the unique characteristics of its school so that, ultimately, the improvement plan recommended is a good fit and not simply a replication of the approach used in the other school.

CHAPTER SUMMARY

The rationale is compelling for school counselors to collect data relevant to school counseling programs and guidelines for developing data-driven comprehensive school counseling programs. School counselors need to embrace the use of data in the course of their daily work for a number of reasons. Most important, counselors in schools must be able to demonstrate how counseling makes a difference in successful educational outcomes for students. With this type of data, school counselors can show others the important contributions to student academic success of a carefully planned school counseling program. The data encourage the counselor when there are successful results and provide useful feedback when the results do not hit the mark.

School reform efforts are best documented with carefully chosen outcome measures that provide clear indicators of academic success. Such measures assist the school counselor in communicating results in a straightforward and understandable manner. Stakeholders appreciate such proactive approaches to accountability within schools. The best way for school counselors to be proactively accountable is to be involved with data collection and analysis and then "let the data speak."

REVIEW AND REFLECT

1. Arrange a visit with a local school counselor to review the school district's data systems (usually available online). Explain that you are a school counseling graduate student learning about what information is available and how it is used. Ask the counselor to show you how he/she accesses some of the important school data described in this chapter, for example, attendance rates, dropout rates, and failure rates. Ask if there are specific target areas that are the focus for change that were identified through the school data system. Ask if there are specific programs in place for systems change and what type of data are being collected to demonstrate the outcome. Share what you learned in a small group.

2. Interview a district coordinator of school counselors and ask the following questions while taking notes.
   a. Describe the geographical location of the school district and unique features of the area.

   _____

   _____

   _____

   _____

   b. What is the total number of students the district serves? _____
   c. How many schools are there at each level within the school district?

_____

_____

_____

_____

_____

   d. How many alternative schools are there? _____
   e. Is there a district-wide developmental counseling program?
       _____ Yes _____ No
       If yes, please describe.

_____

_____

_____

_____

_____

_____

_____

   f. Does the counseling program incorporate the ASCA National Model and
       Standards?   _____ Yes _____ No
   g. Do the district school counselors meet regularly?   _____ Yes _____ No
   h. How would you describe the current state of school counseling in the
       district?

_____

_____

_____

_____

_____

_____

_____

_____

i. How are school counselors viewed in the school district? by students? parents? teachers? administration? support staff?

_____

_____

_____

_____

_____

_____

_____

_____

_____

_____

_____

_____

_____

_____

_____

_____

_____

_____

3. Summarize your interview for exercise 2 in a class, including the numerical information, and in a discussion compare your results with the results obtained by other students.

RELEVANT WEBSITES

American School Counselor Association: www.schoolcounselor.org
The Education Trust: www.edtrust.org
Research Made Easy: www.questia.com
Research Monographs: http://www.cscor.org/Research_Monographs.htm
U.S. Department of Education: www.ed.gov
Phi Delta Kappa International: www.pdkintl.org
American Educational Research Association: www.AERA.net
Northeastern Educational Research Association: www.NERA-education.org

REFERENCES

American School Counselor Association. (2003). *The ASCA national model: A framework for school counseling programs*. Alexandria, VA: Author.

Atkinson, D. R., Furlong, M., & Janoff, D. S. (1979). A four-component model for proactive accountability in school counseling. *School Counselor, 26*, 222–228.

Fairchild, T. N. (1986). Time analysis: Accountability tool for counselors. *School Counselor, 34*, 36–43.

Gysbers, N. C., Lapan, R. T., & Blair, M. (1999). Closing in on statewide implementation of a comprehensive guidance program model. *Professional School Counseling, 2*, 357–366.

Krumboltz, J. D. (1974). An accountability model for counselors. *Personnel and Guidance Journal, 52*, 639–646.

Schmidt, J. J. (2003). *Counseling in schools*. Boston: Allyn and Bacon.

Tucker, S. (1996). *Benchmarking: A guide for educators*. Thousand Oaks, CA: Corwin Press.

CHAPTER 12

Next Step: Walking the Walk of Leadership

THE WISDOM OF THE ASCA NATIONAL STANDARDS AND NATIONAL MODEL

Andrea had been a school counselor at the middle school level for four years. During her first two years working as a school counselor, she simply followed the directives of the autocratic administrator for whom she worked and her school guidance program primarily reflected the administrator's agenda for the school. As she continued in her career, she became convinced that to best meet the needs of all students, her school guidance program should align itself with the ASCA National Standards (Campbell & Dahir, 1997) and the ASCA National Model (2003). By the time a more democratic administrator who believed in shared leadership was assigned to her school in her third year as a school counselor, Andrea saw herself as a new-vision counselor. She obtained the school administrator's support to build a results-based school counseling program. This comprehensive developmental approach to school counseling was in contrast to the approach used in the other schools in her district and other districts in her city which provided traditional mental health and crisis-response services. As she conscientiously followed the ASCA National Model, incorporating the ASCA National Standards, she questioned counselors in other schools and districts in her city about why they were not embracing the ASCA model and standards. They explained that although they knew about and approved of the ASCA model and standards, they did not have the time for the additional work required.

As she engaged in discussion with the other counselors, Andrea recalled that she had felt the same way early in her career as a middle school counselor. During her first years in the profession when she simply followed the administrator's agenda, she could not imagine fitting even one additional responsibility into her schedule. However, it had not taken Andrea long to realize that her job description was not clear, and that the administrators, teachers, staff, students, and parents did not understand what she did. For that matter, she was confused much of the time herself. When she simply followed her administrator's direction without questioning the agenda she sacrificed much of the comprehensive school counseling plan that was a vital part of her role in support of the school mission.

For example, because she was a certified teacher, the principal frequently asked her to substitute for teachers who called in sick. Teachers sought her help in disciplining children, especially a specific group of disruptive boys. Andrea was given the responsibility of running the snack bar during lunch to help raise money for necessary school materials not supplied in the budget. She prepared and mailed out report cards for all students. She and the other counselor at the school were responsible for creating the master schedule for students. On occasion, she even had to fill in for the principal and the school nurse.

During those early years as a school counselor, Andrea felt pulled in many directions. Her education had prepared her well for school counseling in the 21st century. Her professors in graduate school inspired her with the vision developed by ASCA and the Education Trust and informed her about what to expect as she entered the profession. However, she wasn't quite prepared for the barriers to comprehensive developmental guidance that she faced on a daily basis. None of her professors or school supervisors had prepared her for the discrepancy between her educational preparation and her actual role as a school counselor. The barriers raised Andrea's awareness of the risk of slow burnout in the chosen profession for which she had such great passion.

Case Discussion

Questions About This Case

- What were some of the key issues that this school counselor faced?
- What options did she have for coping with the reality of her position as a school counselor?
- How can a school counselor develop the resiliency to survive and thrive in a demanding profession?
- What messages about school counselor roles and priorities does this scenario convey?
- What can we learn from this case example about working with the administration in a school?

Further Thoughts on This Case

If Andrea was convinced that she needed to take a leadership role in order to initiate the systems change needed at her school and in her district, she could find allies in other counselors in the school district who wanted to see their roles in the schools transformed to align with the vision at the national level. And, if she thought about the costs of taking a stand for her profession and decided that it was worth the risk, she could choose to lead her district counselors toward getting the change in motion.

At her school, she could make a commitment to develop and promote a comprehensive competency-based school counseling program, guided by the ASCA National Model. This task would require her to be assertive with those who tried to change her role without considering the impact on the guidance program. She could add some members to her small school counseling program advisory council. The new members recruited should be more vocal advocates for school counseling than the current members. She could request that the principal of her school meet with her on a regular basis to review goals and progress and provide input into the comprehensive competency-based school counseling program. She could also ask the principal to attend specific school counseling advisory council meetings.

Andrea could also take an active role on relevant district committees and in her state professional school counselors' association. By accepting these leadership positions, Andrea would be increasing the demands on her time and energy. However, her involvement would likely result in the support she needed from other educational leaders and the other school counselors in her district for the challenges ahead.

CHAPTER OBJECTIVES

The objectives of this chapter are to:

1. Integrate key concepts from the ASCA National Model into the mission of school counselors.
2. Describe how the ASCA National Model realistically translates into daily practice for school counselors.
3. Emphasize the importance of the school counselor leadership skills that have been presented and discussed in previous chapters.

THE MISSION OF SCHOOL COUNSELORS AND THE NATIONAL MODEL

According to ASCA National Standards (Campbell & Dahir, 1997), the purpose of school counseling programs is to promote and enhance learning, and the goal is to enable all students to become successful, contributing members of society. The National Standards identify the competencies expected of all students as indicators of their school performance. School counselors are encouraged to use a collaborative leadership approach to develop, implement, monitor, and adjust the comprehensive school counseling program.

School counselor leaders can use the ASCA National Model workbook (2004) as a guide to implementing the ASCA National Model in their school. The guidelines include starting with the existing school counseling program, allowing for minor adaptations for a specific school, using a team approach, expecting some staff resistance, being flexible, not reinventing the wheel, and cooperating with teachers.

Aligning the School Mission Statement

When starting with an existing program, the school counselor should lead by approaching various stakeholders of the school's guidance program to invite their involvement and input. The group needs to review the philosophy and mission statements of the state department of education, the school district, and the school as well as any existing guidance philosophy and mission statements at each level. The philosophy and mission statements of the school should align with the state's and district's guidance philosophy and mission statement. For assistance in developing a new philosophy and mission statement, school counselors and stakeholders can consult the ASCA National Model section on the foundation for guidelines.

In order to ensure that the philosophy and mission statements are truly "owned" by the school community and guide activities throughout the system, their development should be a team effort, actively involving key stakeholders. The mission statement should be action oriented. See Chapter 10 for a discussion of the process of developing a mission statement for a school.

Educating Stakeholders About the National Standards

The school counselor as educational leader needs to be familiar with the ASCA National Standards for students and prepared to educate the stakeholders regarding them. The national standards are another critical component of the foundation for a comprehensive developmental guidance plan. These standards identify and organize the knowledge and skills that a comprehensive school counseling program must transmit to all students. The guidance plan should be aligned with the National Standards, including the three domains (academic, career, and personal/social) and the three standards for each domain with associated competencies and the corresponding indicators for each competency.

Box 12-1 provides a summary of the domains and the standards. The complete National Standards, including the 124 competencies and associated indicators, are included in the National Model. School counselors are responsible for the leadership activities of planning, organizing, and coordinating a school counseling program each year and for ensuring that students achieve the competencies over the course of their K–12 education.

SCHOOL COUNSELOR LEADERS AS EFFECTIVE COMMUNICATORS

School counselors as educational leaders must be excellent communicators. In order to establish effective school counseling programs, they must educate administrators, teachers, parents, and others about what school counseling is and how the school's comprehensive developmental guidance program relates directly to the academic success of students. They must demonstrate how counseling standards support state standards and school improvement goals. The ASCA (2004) website offers the following tips for school counselors to keep in mind when working with the school administration and local boards of education:

- Focus on student results, not what counselors do.
- Data speak louder than words. Use charts and graphs to show results.

Box 12-1   Domains and Standards of the National Standards for School Counseling Programs

Academic Development	*Standard A:* Students will acquire the attitudes, knowledge, and skills that contribute to effective learning in school across the life span.
	Standard B: Students will complete school with the academic preparation essential to choosing from a wide range of postsecondary options, including college.
	Standard C: Students will understand the relationship of academics to the world of work and to life at home in the community.
Career Development	*Standard A:* Students will acquire the skills to investigate the world of work in relation to knowledge of self and to make informed career decisions.
	Standard B: Students will employ strategies to achieve future career success and satisfaction.
	Standard C: Students will understand the relationship among personal qualities, education and training, and the world of work.
Personal/Social Development	*Standard A:* Students will acquire the attitudes, knowledge, and interpersonal skills to help them understand and respect themselves and others.
	Standard B: Students will make decisions, set goals, and take necessary action to achieve goals.
	Standard C: Students will understand safety and survival skills.

Adapted from Campbell & Dahir, 1997.

- Build a booster club, better known as an advisory council, who will speak on your behalf at board meetings.
- Ask a successful student to speak on behalf of school counselors and follow his/her success story with numbers representing success with many students. For example, have a 19- or 20-year-old student tell the board how if it weren't for the school counselor he/she would not be in college. Follow this up with a chart showing the percentage increase of students attending a four-year university over the last three years due in part to the efforts of the counselor.
- No matter what your administration proposes in cuts, it is the local school board that must approve them. Lobby the board; for example, take board members to lunch. You, the community, elected the board members to represent you. Let them know what you want.
- Become politically active in community affairs.
- Frame the school counseling program as an investment in the students in your school.
- The board presentation is like an annual dividend meeting demonstrating the return on investment in student results.

When designing a comprehensive school counseling program, the school counselor needs to strategically invite diverse representation from students, parents, teachers, counselors, administrators, and the community to participate on the school counseling advisory council. The advisory council demonstrates the emphasis on team effort immediately after the program begins. The focus of the council is to review the school counseling program, including its goals and results, and to make recommendations to the school counselor or counseling department. While developing the school counseling program with the assistance of the advisory council, the school counselor must make some adaptations for the unique needs and characteristics of their specific school. The school counselor, principal, and advisory council work as a team on behalf of the school counseling program, supporting it as it meets the needs of all students.

Coping with Resistance

School counselor leaders who initiate transformation of their programs should expect some staff resistance. In some schools and school districts, this can be an understatement. There are school districts that not only do not subscribe to the National Model but do not subscribe to any form of comprehensive school counseling model. These districts continue to respond primarily to individual student needs, focusing mainly on the gifted and at-risk students. This approach leaves the needs of the rest of the school population unaddressed in any systematic way. School counselor educational leaders who function as change agents realize that systemic change takes time, along with persistent effort to work through the resistance.

School counselors, especially those with programs under construction, need to be flexible and creative. It is important to anticipate the unanticipated. In other words, the effective comprehensive school counseling plan should allow some room for adjustment and revision based on changing school needs. We live in an environment of rapid change, and although we cannot predict the future we can anticipate that change will occur. Change is a given. School counselors and their advisory councils can be flexible and creative in allowing for the impact of change within the school environment.

School counselors as educational leaders in the 21st century do not need to reinvent the wheel. The ASCA National Model, the ASCA website, many other school counseling–related websites, model programs, school districts, departments of education, and numerous other resources exist to support the work of school counselors. Many materials, including curriculum materials, are free and available online. Counselors can adapt these materials as needed for a particular population in a specific school. School counselor leaders know how to work smarter instead of harder by effectively utilizing the myriad of resources at their disposal.

Maintaining Cooperative and Collaborative Relationships

School counselor leaders use their interpersonal skills to develop and maintain cooperative and collaborative relationships with teachers in the learning community of the school. As educational leaders, they strategically align their counseling program's mission with the mission of the school. Therefore, school counselors and teachers have a common mission pointing to common goals that lead to student academic success. They are most successful in achieving such goals when they collaborate in the interest of all students. The unique training of school counselors prepares them well to be skillful facilitators of cooperative and collaborative relationships with teachers and others in learning communities.

Self-Assessment and Exploration

In this exercise you will practice promoting your school counseling program using some basic public relations tools.

Instructions: Following some of the ASCA (2004) guidelines for promoting school counseling with administrators and board members, develop a brief presentation and an accompanying brochure about a specific school counseling program. The school can be one in which you completed a practicum or an internship. You can develop a PowerPoint® or overhead transparency presentation demonstrating the relationship between the school guidance program and student results. Remember to use charts and graphs. Use quotations from students and consider samples of outstanding student work or lists of achievements. Share your presentation with your learning group.

PROGRAM DEVELOPMENT

The school counselor leader can also use the National Model workbook as a resource to guide the stakeholders' steps for school counseling program development. The specific steps outlined in the workbook include: planning and leadership designation, building the foundation, designing the delivery system, setting up the school counseling program, working with the school counseling program, promoting the school counseling program, monitoring program results, monitoring students' progress, and making the transition. Each of the steps for program development will be explored to provide clarification.

Effective school counseling programs require planning and designation of leadership in order to assure that goals will be set, actions will be taken, data will be collected and analyzed, and outcomes will be evaluated. The school counselor as educational leader ensures that the required planning and leadership designation occurs on behalf of the school counseling program. Evaluation of program outcomes leads to decision making by the counselor, administrators, and advisory council regarding whether changes are needed to improve outcomes. The school counselor's skilled leadership behaviors that facilitate team planning and his/her designation of leadership keep the cycle of accountability in motion so that a school counseling program continuously improves.

By building a strong foundation, the school counselor and program stakeholders prepare the way for the construction of a meaningful and systematic program that addresses the needs and promotes the success of all students. The foundation includes the common values shared by the stakeholders of the school, the philosophy of the school, and the school's mission statement. The school counselor as leader in the development of these elements of the foundation can effectively engage others in the process by encouraging careful reflection, discussion, and consensus building of the key stakeholders in the school.

When a solid foundation is established for a school counseling program, the construction crew (counselor, administrators, and advisory council) can safely proceed with designing the delivery system. The school counselor leader guides this process by assuring that it addresses the priorities set in the foundation by developing action

Table 12-1   School Counseling Master Calendar

Maldonado Elementary School, School Year: 2005–2006	
August Counselor orientation	*January* Diversity Problem-solving skills
September Academic skills and goals	*February* Career pathways and goal setting Decision-making process
October Drug and gang awareness Red ribbon week	*March* Test-taking support and strategies
November Disability awareness	*April* Peer pressure
December Getting along: bullying, friendship, conflict resolution, and feelings	*May* Transition from elementary to middle school Goal setting for 2006–2007

Suarez, 2004.

plans with time allotments for components, choosing a guidance curriculum, forging agreements on who performs which activities, identifying the type of data to be collected to evaluate program effectiveness, and obtaining administrative support.

When the school counselor(s), administrators, and advisers ensure that there is equal access to the program, an adequate budget and resources, a collaborative approach, state leadership, and technical support, and when all required documentation is completed, the school counselor educational leader can put the counseling program into place and manage it. In leading the program, the school counselor implements the school counseling curriculum at all grades and follows the calendars and master school counseling schedule. Table 12-1 is an example of a school counseling master calendar for an elementary school. Box 12-2 provides an example of a lesson plan for first grade in the same elementary school.

In order to promote the school counseling program and to advocate for it and for the school counseling profession, the counselor as educational leader develops a program brochure and presents it to the school staff and the school board. The counselor can also send the brochure to students' homes and distribute it at meetings in the community to showcase the program. In addition to distributing a brochure, schools are strongly encouraged to develop their own website with a counseling section used to communicate with and educate parents, students, faculty, administrators, and other visitors to the website about the school counseling program and counseling-related issues.

Box 12-2   First-Grade Guidance Lesson Plan for Maldonado Elementary School

---

TUSD Classroom Guidance Lesson Plan/Evaluation

Counselor Name	Zulema Suarez
School	Maldonado Elementary School
Title of Lesson	Helping Hands
Quarter	Third
Grade Level	First
Time Required	30 minutes
Number of Students	23
ASCA National Standards	

- PS-A2.6: Use effective communications skills
- PS-A2.7: Know that communication involves speaking, listening, and nonverbal behavior
- PS-B1.1: Use decision-making and problem-solving model
- PS-B1.3: Identify alternative solutions to a problem
- PS-C1.6: Identify resource people in the school and community, and know how to seek their help

Competency Addressed   Demonstrate skills in resolving conflicts with peers and adults

Activity   Pretest activity

Review each finger on the "Helping Hand" with examples of how the people can help (family person, teacher/principal, nurse/doctor, friend, and counselor/social worker). The students then color each finger.

Script (use flexibly)   I have come into your classroom today to tell you about myself and what I do here at school. I am the school counselor, a school helper. Everybody in the world needs help sometimes. Even I need to ask for help. Sometimes I need to ask the principal or teachers for help. (Give examples of people you have asked for help and how they helped.) Can any of you think of a time when you helped someone? (Let the children give you examples of whom they have helped and how. Reinforce the idea that everybody needs help sometimes. Pass out the Helping Hand handout.)

There are lots of people you can go to for help. Let's talk about some of those helping people. (Give a scenario for each person on your fingers, starting with the pinky. Allow them to answer. Have them follow along with each finger.) If you were thirsty at home and you couldn't reach the cups, whom could you ask for help? (Allow different answers.) Good, those are family members at home who can help you when you have problems. (Do this for all fingers, but not the thumb.)

All of these people we have talked about are helping people, and I am a helping person, too! (Give examples of things school counselors help children with as well as the things school counselors do at school. Ask the children to take out their

(continued)

Box 12-2	*(continued)*
	green crayon.) I would like everyone to color the thumb on the helping hand green. The reason why we colored just the thumb green is because I want all of you to remember you can always go to your school counselor if you have a problem. Your teacher can be a good helper with a problem, but your teacher has a lot of children in the class and may not be able to talk with you as much as they would like. That's why a teacher might ask me talk with you.
Evaluation	Pretest question: "Who are the helping hands in your life?" Posttest question: "Who are the helping hands in your life?"
Materials/Resources	A copy of the "Helping Hand" (a drawing of a hand with the categories of helpers listed above with one per finger and the school counselor on the thumb).

School counselors as educational leaders recognize that a system for monitoring program results and students' progress is critical to demonstrating that school counseling programs make a difference to the academic success of students. School counselors and their program advisors must choose indicators of student success carefully and choose more than one indicator.

From the point at which a school considers transformation of the school counseling program and alignment with the National Model, through the decision and actual transition, the school counselor as proactive change agent must help the stakeholders see that the initial investment of time and effort required will be worth the cost. The school counselor as educational leader and others involved in the reconstruction process will need patience to see the process through, persistence to stay the course with each step of the change agenda, creative processing to see ways past resistance and other barriers, openness to new ideas and diverse perspectives of other stakeholders, and a willingness to take risks and to trust others.

When the comprehensive school counseling program is in place, the school counselor as educational leader and stakeholders face the task of maintaining and continuously improving it. They will need to monitor program outcome results and indicators of student success for evidence that either supports the current approach or suggests a need for an alternative approach.

This is a good point at which to review the list of leadership characteristics of the integrated model of school counselor leadership proposed in Chapter 3. Consider how the following behaviors and characteristics were demonstrated in the material in this and previous chapters. School counselors as educational leaders do the following:

- Develop their own leadership from within based on their values and the principles by which they live.
- Live with integrity and demonstrate character and morality by doing the right thing instead of being overly concerned with doing things right.

- Listen to their own inner voice. They reject superficial efforts at school transformation including slogans and numerical quotas without the foundation of a moral imperative.
- Learn by experience, engaging in reflection as they develop as leaders, continually growing as self-directed adult learners who use a whole-brain approach as they process information.
- Value and promote harmonious relationships and see leadership as a way to serve others and to develop a sense of belonging. They demonstrate cultural competence and value, nurture, and celebrate differences and social interest in their daily lives. They advocate for social justice.
- Model a democratic way of supporting the ASCA guiding vision by sharing leadership opportunities and encouraging others to make contributions to the learning community that provide a sense of belonging and experience of power, freedom, and fun.
- Believe in collaboration and are skilled in developing strategic alliances and contracts that facilitate support and cooperation. They seek the right mentors who have positive values and philosophies.
- Facilitate conditions of trust, open and effective communication, and opportunities for positive growth and self-actualization. They do this by demonstrating congruence, empathy, and unconditional positive regard.
- Are followers first, and believe in a guiding vision that is associated with mental pictures.
- Share a commitment with other educational leaders to the school's guiding vision and constancy of purpose in transformation of the school with a clear sense of the future.
- View life as an adventure, life as a career; take active risks; seek challenges; demonstrate passion for life with curiosity and daring.
- Stay current in their field and engage in continual growth, learning by experience using a whole-brain approach, mental pictures, self-direction, innovation, and origination, seeking full self-expression and self-actualization.
- Thrive on change and challenging the status quo, asking what and why.
- Utilize systems thinking and develop strategic alliances and interdependent relationships that promote the school's guiding vision.
- Skillfully obtain support and cooperation and use contracts that support accountability and responsibility in achieving measurable goals and collecting objective data.

CHAPTER SUMMARY

Currently school counselors are charged with integrating key concepts from the National Model into their mission and with determining how the model realistically translates into daily practice. The leadership characteristics, skills, models, and styles presented in this book provide a conceptual framework for school counselors developing as educational leaders. The various leadership roles expected of school counselors can be better understood and articulated within this framework.

Tying the ASCA National Model to school counselor daily practice requires educational leadership skills to ensure effectiveness. Practical resources such as the National Model workbook which contains steps for school counseling program development are available to guide school counselor leaders and their collaborators. School counselors lead, advocate, and collaborate with other stakeholders on a daily basis in order to meet the challenge of turning the vision of the National Model into a reality in our schools.

REVIEW AND REFLECT

1. Either on your own or in a small group, brainstorm the possible objections of school personnel to the transformation of a school counseling program to align with the National Model. How would you respond to those objections in order to help others understand the need for and the benefits of a comprehensive school counseling program with all components of the National Model? Note some of the key responses in your leadership journal for later reference as needed.
2. Which roles of a school counselor will be most challenging to you? What leadership skills will you use to meet these challenges? Include these in your leadership plan, if they are not already included.

RELEVANT WEBSITES

American School Counselor Association: www.schoolcounselor.org
Association for Supervision and Curriculum Development: www.ascd.org
Reviews of educational policies and practices effective in closing the achievement gap: www.ed.gov/databases/ERIC_Digests/ed460191.html
The Education Trust: www.edtrust.org
The International Center for Leadership in Education: www.daggett.com/
The School Leadership Development Unit: www.sofweb.vic.edu.au/pd/schlead/
http://21stcenturyschools.northcarolina.edu/center

REFERENCES

American School Counselor Association. (2003). *The ASCA national model: A framework for school counseling programs*. Alexandria, VA: Author.

American School Counselor Association. (2004). *The ASCA national model workbook*. Alexandria, VA: Author.

American School Counselor Association homepage. (2004). Available: www.http://schoolcounselor.org

Campbell, C. A., & Dahir, C. A. (1997). *The national standards for school counseling programs*. Alexandria, VA: American School Counselor Association.

Suarez, Z. (2004). *Comprehensive competency based guidance program notebook*. Unpublished manuscript.

INDEX